Celiac
AND THE
Beast

A LOVE STORY BETWEEN A GLUTEN-FREE GIRL, HER GENES, AND A BROKEN DIGESTIVE TRACT

B

ERICA DERMER

This book contains advice and information relating to health care—and more specifically, management of celiac disease. It is not intended to replace any medical advice and should be used only to supplement regular care by your medical professional. It is recommended that you seek your physician's advice before embarking on any medical program or treatment. The publisher/author disclaims liability for any medical outcomes that may occur as a result of applying information found in this book. Your reliance upon information and content obtained by you in or through this publication is solely at your own risk.

For information about this title or to order other books and/or electronic media, contact the publisher:
Celiac and the Beast
http://www.celiacandthebeast.com
CeliacandtheBeast@gmail.com

ISBN: 978-0-9899574-0-3
Printed in the United States of America
Cover design: Matt Saling
Interior design: 1106 Design

Dedicated to anyone who has ever told me that I could do anything I put my mind to, because this book proves I can! Except become a doctor, because I could never pass organic chemistry, or a trail runner, because the outdoors terrifies me. I also couldn't become an astronaut because of my motion sickness. I guess that includes all travel-related careers too. Basically, this book is dedicated to anyone who ever told me I could write a book. Thanks.

Contents

Introduction: The Gluten-Free Preamble to the Ramble

I wish I could tell you that if I ate a bowl of Pasta Roni right now, I would swiftly crap my pants.

I only wish this because then you would plainly see that something is very, *very* wrong with my insides. But no, unfortunately I can still eat a bowl of Pasta Roni (or any other delicious shitty, cheap pasta meal from a box with little nutritional value) and keep on going like a champion. Only days later would I feel lethargic and bitchy and riddled with anxiety. Days to weeks later I would develop giant sores on the inside of my mouth and on the back of my tongue that would render me speechless and probably crying in my car listening to Sad FM[1]. While this may seem like the diatribe of a crazy person (and sometimes I believe it *might* be), this is just my life with celiac disease.

Most of you probably read the above diatribe and said, "Ugh! Why do I want to read the book of someone who isn't crapping their pants at the mere sight of a pancake like I am?" Well, actually, I *am* just like you.

---

[1] Yes, I just referenced *Bridget Jones's Diary*. This was a pivotal book and movie for my often-single early adulthood. I often thought my first book would be much like it. Too bad I fell in love soon after diagnosis. Oh, fate . . .

While my symptoms may be different from a typical celiac (although, what exactly is *typical* considering that this scallywag of a disease has 300 symptoms[2]), I experience the same life post-gluten as every other celiac—and that's what I'm here for.

Just in case you're not sure about what celiac disease really is, let's give you a refresher course. According to the University of Chicago Celiac Disease Center,

> *"Celiac disease is an inherited autoimmune disease like diabetes or rheumatoid arthritis. Autoimmune means a person's immune system mistakenly attacks one of the body's own tissues or cells. When a person who has celiac disease eats gluten—a protein found in wheat, rye, and barley—the individual's immune system responds by attacking the small intestine and inhibiting the absorption of important nutrients into the body."*

While life with celiac disease or gluten intolerance (now called Non-Celiac Gluten Sensitivity—NCGS) is not a pretty life, it's the only one we have. And while life with celiac disease shouldn't be about smiling, faking it and pretending like rainbows are shooting out of our respective asses, I'm about to make a bold and positive statement about the disease.

Being diagnosed with celiac disease is the best thing that's ever happened to me.

Go ahead; call me a name right now. You're not even doing it behind my back. Just think of the worst name ever and call me that for saying the aforementioned statement. You're probably saying "(expletives deleted) Who does she think she is? This disease has ruined my life, etc."

---

[2] This stat was taken from the University of Chicago Celiac Disease Center, but you can easily see this if you ask every celiac to tell you their incredibly varied symptoms. http://www.cureceliacdisease.org/living-with-celiac/guide/symptoms

Well, it *is* the best thing that has ever happened to me, and I can tell you briefly (although I will provide an in-depth explanation throughout the book) why it is.

1. I finally understand what's wrong with my body
2. My diagnosis gave me a game plan for the rest of my life
3. It's allowed me to meet so many new friends across the country whom I never would have met otherwise
4. It's a litmus test for friendship and relationships
5. It's given me a purpose in life: to educate and advocate

Let me hit you with another bold statement that is also true.

Being diagnosed with celiac disease is the hardest thing that's ever happened to me.

Now, I feel like I've accomplished some cool things in my life that were also pretty difficult. I got my degree from college and graduated with honors. I worked in market research, giving research and development reports to some massive Fortune 500 (and above) clients. I've gone on live TV and once cohosted a show on a major network. I've put myself into therapy before, which is something considering how difficult it is for a Type A personality to admit they aren't perfect. I've fallen in love. I got a tattoo that is now considered seriously regrettable. I started freelancing and didn't know when my next paycheck was coming. I also own a snake.[3] I even started my own website and apparel line with all of my life savings.

But, going gluten free has been my hardest endeavor yet. I always tell my readers that it gets easier—and it does. Everything does. Your brain

---

[3] Seriously, why did no one warn me as a child that I was about to purchase an animal that lives 40-plus years in captivity? You should have to sign a legal document before purchasing an animal that will probably outlive all of your major relationships and purchases.

is a magical creature, and it's really good at homeostasis—regulating processes and maintaining equilibrium. Living gluten free *will* become second nature to you. Everything that is hard now—and everything that makes you want to sit in a corner and cry, possibly crapping your pants or throwing up in your handbag—*well, that will all get easier too.*

It will never get easy—but it will get easier.

However, I believe that things that are hard make you a better person—at least I think I've become a better person because of it. Struggles build your character and make you a badass. Every one of you who survives another day as a celiac is an honorary superhero. So strap on your cape and pat yourself on the back. You are a champion, conquering the wheat-filled world, one gluten-free cupcake at a time.

See, I've already got you thinking about the positive side of this diagnosis. Either that or you already put the book down and are searching for something on television. Might I suggest *Family Guy* reruns?

But listen folks; don't put the book down yet. I mean, you probably purchased it already, so it would be a waste of your money if you stopped now. I promise: there are some really crappy (literally) parts of this disease. It's not easy, so I'm going to give you a lot of real talk—and real stories—that tell you all about my experience with the disease.

And eat that gluten-free cupcake for Christ's sake; it's going to be a bumpy ride.

Disclaimers: Read This Book at Your Own Risk

This book contains opinions! I have opinions—a lot of them actually! The opinions here are my own. There's a good chance that you and I don't have the same taste (in products, food, favorite travel spots, men, etc.), so please make sure you take my writing that way. Just as on my website, if our opinions differ, I'm totally cool with that. I'm not saying that it's "my way or the highway" when it comes to living gluten free. Everyone can have a different perspective, unless your perspective includes cheating with gluten, and then it's *not* cool! This book is about my thoughts and perspectives on living a gluten-free life. If you prefer the musings of Elisabeth Hasselbeck, go for it; she has plenty of books out, and I've read them and enjoyed most of them.

Opinions are like buttholes: everyone has one. I just happen to like mine the best. But enough about buttholes. . . .

This book is based on my memory, faulty as it may be. While I'm not writing a straightforward memoir, it's been a tough five years, and I'm retelling the story to the best of my abilities. Luckily, Facebook helped me chronicle my symptoms, so I have a written diary of when I started to feel like doggie doo-doo. If things are off on timing, hey, I'm human. And I'm really happy that my brain functions as well as it does now after all of the medication I've had to take to get here. What's my name again? Where do I live?

With the amount of brain fog that I'm sure you've encountered, I'm sure you understand.

It also contains some f&$%ing swearing. Sometimes I swear.[4] I've done it since I was a kid. I've never been a prim and proper lady; I've always been more like a sassy lady truck driver you might see on TV. That's just what makes me who I am. The English language is great, and it's given me plenty of opportunities to use the thesaurus and find words that I struggle to replace for swear words. Sometimes it's just not as effective to say that "gluten is just so ding-dang rude!" I feel that "gluten is an *asshole*" really gets the point across better. Although the former is kind of adorable when you say it with a Southern accent.

There are some swear words in this book, because I wanted to write it like I was sitting with you in your living room, giving you the low-down about the disease.

Ch-ch-changes happen without my knowledge! Some brands and ingredients may be different than when I last talked about them. Maybe the company hikes up the prices or maybe the brand is discontinued. When I wrote this book, it was the summer of 2013. Flying cars had not been invented yet, but I have high hopes for 2014. If you're reading this after it's been written, there's a chance that something has changed. Who knows? Maybe I'm a blonde now.

If you're looking for a product that I talk about in this book, please take your health into your own hands and check the current ingredients, gluten-free certification, etc.

---

[4] This may be the biggest understatement of the entire book. Like when I go for blood work and the nurse asks me if I've done this before.

Not yet a doctor, but maybe one day! Sometimes people ask me medical questions concerning gluten-free living or being a celiac. I am not a doctor. I think Dr. Dermer even sounds weird. Perhaps Doctor CeliacBeast is better. I've never played a doctor on TV or even in the theater. Nothing in this book or on my website is a professional medical opinion; they're simply personal opinions based on what I've gone through as a celiac. Always consult a real medical professional if you have health concerns or issues about your gluten-free diet. And always consult a doctor before altering your diet—especially before "going gluten free!" I have a great doctor at Mayo Clinic if you're willing to travel!

The statements contained on my website or in this book have not been evaluated by the Food and Drug Administration—or my mom for that matter. I'm not responsible for your health, but *you* definitely should be!

My Celiac—Not Yours, but Still Awesome

I've now blogged about being a celiac for a year and a half. If I have learned anything in this short time, it's that every celiac is different and unique—like a goddamn snowflake. When people ask me what happens when I eat gluten, they suspect that I have raging diarrhea or feel incredibly sick. Nope; in fact, when I was served an entire plate of regular pasta, I ate the whole thing,[5] and my body did nothing out of the ordinary to warn me that I shouldn't have. I don't have the built-in alarm that many celiacs have—that sometimes-instant, but definitely quick, reaction to gluten. Even cross-contamination of gluten-free food instantly warns these celiacs that they've eaten poison. Their bodies are quick to react—even within a few hours. God, a few hours is like lightning speed compared to how my body reacts.

Since I don't get the bellyaching, nauseated, crampy craps like others, I get to sit and wait days, or even weeks, for my symptoms to surface. I haven't really timed my symptoms out, although I'm halfway tempted to eat a "real" cookie and then journal my symptoms for days to see

---

[5] There's more on that story later. Spoiler alert—it doesn't end well.

exactly how long it takes for me to react. By "halfway" I mean it would be an excuse to eat a Dunkin' Donuts pink frosted donut again—*for science of course.*

But, I won't because that would really suck. I'd much rather save those days of misery for when some crappy server messes up my order and I have someone to yell at for how I feel besides myself.

So what exactly *does* happen to me when I eat gluten? Strangers always ask me how I found out that I had celiac disease. As an atypical celiac, it's hard to explain because my symptoms are so different than the "typical" digestive ones[6]. And therefore, diagnosis came a little harder to me than to others, who may complain of violent illness as soon as the culprit is ingested.

I turn into the Incredible Hulk of Hot Messes when glutened. I am a ravenous bitch, but at the same time, a crazy anxiety-filled train wreck. Although it's not apparent to me, it sure is apparent to other people. My dude likes to brag that he knows when I've been glutened before I do just because I turn into a bitch. Although sometimes I think that the people closest to me assume I'm like that normally.

My joints hurt. My bones hurt. My muscles hurt. My body hurts. All I want to do all day is sleep. And although most people would think that it's super fun to sleep all day, I feel like the only thing I can do is breathe, eat, and watch Netflix. I don't feel well enough to go work out and have to push myself with anything that requires energy besides drinking wine and scrounging for chocolate in my cupboards.

Most prevalently, my tongue swells up and I develop large aphthous ulcers[7] on the inside of my mouth or on my tongue. These are incredibly painful; I can barely eat or drink without sharp pain, and it lasts for a week or more. On top of that, my speech becomes slurred—which is

---

[6] I always thought I was an asymptomatic celiac, but as time progressed, I realized that I just didn't have the typical digestive symptoms. I had a whole set of impressive symptoms outside my intestines that were a total pain in my proverbial ass.

[7] Aphthous stomatitis ulcers are like canker sores on crack. They reoccur whenever I ingest gluten and are one of my only outward tale-tell signs of being glutened.

always awesome when you're giving client presentations for work. Ain't nothing like sounding drunk or incoherent to someone who just paid your company thousands of dollars to write a report. "Johnson, who is this train wreck that company ABC has on the line? She sounds like the drug abuser on that reality TV show. Someone should fire her." During the call, I inevitably end up drooling or biting my lip or tongue right on the sore—which is fine because I do my conference calls from home in my pajamas anyways.

I just feel lousy when gluten is involved. I know that it's not really a great description of a symptom, but I think most of you will understand. It's so hard to put a descriptor on it.

That's what happens after I get glutened when I have been one hundred percent gluten free for a long period of time. But what symptoms led me to get diagnosed?

That's a *bit* more complicated.

One night after drinking a bottle of wine with my lady friends in 2009, I started feeling awful. I didn't know if it was the wine[8], the bruschetta that I had for dinner, or just a bug. But after that night, I just didn't get better. I had consistent stomach pain and was so nauseated. Not wanting to live with those symptoms for much longer, I hurriedly visited my primary-care physician.

At first, I was diagnosed with an ulcer. Or should I say that I was diagnosed with what they *thought* was an ulcer based on my symptoms. I was put on Sucralfate (also known as carafate suspension or "pink goo"). It's supposed to be soothing to your stomach and/or ulcer, help heal an ulcer, and aid in healing gastritis. The goo forms a barrier so your stomach can heal. Unfortunately, my stomach wasn't the key problem. So although it was super fun to drink pink liquid goo before each meal, it didn't help (you know, since I had celiac disease instead).

---

[8]   I had a lot of wine that night. I had my typical few glasses at dinner (because who doesn't love wine with Italian food). But then when I went home, I opened up another bottle for myself. I *love* wine. But, alas, I cannot blame wine for this issue—unlike other issues like drunk dialing.

On top of the goo, I was given a topical anti-inflammatory for my joints because it felt like I had arthritis. Apparently my body loved being more than one kind of sick all at the same time. When I bought a new IKEA couch in 2009, I distinctly remember sitting on the floor and trying to stuff the cushions and pillows. It was nearly impossible; my joints hurt so badly I had to have my fifty-five-year-old mother do it. It was depressing, and I knew that something wasn't right.

Meanwhile, I was also suffering from debilitating situational anxiety (as opposed to general "I'm terrified of everything" anxiety). I had a Xanax prescription just in case the world got too hard for me to handle. Little did I know I'd need this prescription for years, to get through the rigors of guessing what the hell was wrong with me.

If you're familiar with celiac disease, then you know that all of these symptoms could have been attributed to one disease. However, at the time, it just seemed like I was going through all sorts of bodily shenanigans that were seemingly unrelated. I really wish that I could have put all of the puzzle pieces together sooner.

To put the icing on the cake, I was given all sorts of food sensitivity tests, and they first suggested a gluten-free test diet to "just see" if I felt better and if it helped to tame my beastly stomach and its apparent "wheat sensitivity" (even thought it was—shockingly—a low sensitivity). I gave the new diet a half-assed attempt because they didn't really say that it was important for me to do it with 100% effort. Again, it was all a guessing game at this point. This is also another reason why I'm so passionate about early testing—to avoid the game I went through!

Some older Facebook posts reminded me of how much I struggled back then with the gluten-free diet, even if it was a half-assed version of the lifestyle I currently lead.

> *"Officially hit my gluten-free wall. I'm so irritable and am just over obsessing over everything I eat!"*

"Dear Ulcer Dr., I wish you had better news. Bummed you want me to do GF and special diet for 30 days and are running every allergy test in the book."

Sound familiar? I was such a crybaby when I first went gluten free!

As time progressed and nothing made me feel myself again, I added a gastroenterologist into the mix. While I love my primary-care physician, she could only guess so much before the reinforcements were brought in.

As the mystery unraveled further, I was put on a PPI—a proton-pump inhibitor for my newly diagnosed GERD (gastroesophageal reflux disease). It was supposed to help the acid in my stomach so I wouldn't be burping up bile and feel like I was having an acid baby with all of my food coming back up. I was again told to go on a gluten-free diet to see if it helped. Granted, I still didn't really know what a gluten-free diet entailed so I was just kind of faking it. Again, there was no detailed debriefing on what a gluten-free lifestyle was—just the basics of avoiding a list of certain foods. Oh yeah, it's that easy, right?

When things didn't get better and no test was really definitive, they started questioning everything. At this point they thought it was my gallbladder. I had several consults with a surgeon after numerous gallbladder HIDA scans to measure its effectiveness. One test was super low, and one test was normal. The surgeon was hesitant to take my gallbladder out (and now I'm thankful he didn't). Because we didn't know what it was, I was given a prescription mixture that I had to take after every meal to help my gallbladder—even though we know it wasn't my gallbladder after all. Spoiler alert!

After being on PPIs for a while and taking various random medications every few weeks, I was fed up thinking that I would have no answers for why I just "got sick" and stayed that way. I hate masking my symptoms; I'd rather play detective and figure out what is really wrong. I didn't want to live my whole life not knowing what was going on inside of me. I'd like to think that I have a good relationship with my body, and I wanted to know its secrets. So I got off of my medication, and we sought to find out what was *really* wrong with me. Let's move onto the next diagnosis, shall we?

We next tried numerous annoying gastric-emptying studies and countless radiological exposures. I ate radioactive oatmeal more times than I care to remember.[9] Based on these studies, I was finally diagnosed with gastroparesis. Gastroparesis is a motility disorder caused by the nerves in your stomach not functioning right. I tell people that someone shut off the power grid to my stomach, and it had a really hard time rebooting when it was turned back on. The vagus nerve that told my stomach when it should pump and digest my food was really slow. Therefore, my food would sit in my stomach undigested for long periods of time, leading to chronic fullness, nausea, and feeling awful *all* of the time. Especially when trying to work out on a spin bike without vomiting. Goodbye fresh fruits and veggies and hello to soft food!

I was given Reglan, which is black-boxed by the FDA for causing involuntary and permanent muscle spasms. As I am someone who always gets a rare side effect from medication, I was terrified to take this medication. I was watching my every move to see if anything improved and to notice what was happening to my body. Sure enough, a few days later, I got the shakes. I almost fell asleep on the road driving home because the medication made me so tired. So I went ahead and discontinued *that* one.

I was given a prescription for Domperidone, or "Motilium" which helps with gastric motility. The only issue? Well, it's banned in the US. However, it's available in any other country and is even used as an after-dinner "oh boy I ate too much!" drug that is even advertised on television. But of course I couldn't get prescribed a *normal* drug.

---

[9] Looking back, I find it absurd that they served me oatmeal during the gastric-emptying studies—as the oatmeal was instant oats. Any celiac knows that those oats are contaminated, and I'm sure it triggered celiac symptoms every time I went in for a test. No wonder I still felt like crap regularly. If you have this test, ask for radioactive eggs instead. If you can't have eggs, I have no idea what else they can make radioactive—but I wouldn't hesitate bringing my own gluten-free oats either!

I had to order my new drugs online via an Internet pharmacy. Granted, this one seemed *way* more legitimate than the scams for Viagra I get in my spam mailbox on Gmail, but still it seemed sketchy. Also, these medications routinely get held up in customs, so I never really knew when my medication might arrive. I remember one time I forgot to place an order, and I was left for days without medication. I was too terrified to eat anything larger than a few bites just in case I was sick.

While the medication worked and I felt "better," I didn't really understand what the root of all of my issues was. Like I said, I don't like masking symptoms, so I wanted to know why—out of nowhere—I felt so awful. While I read that gastroparesis could be idiopathic[10], I still wasn't satisfied.

What next? Oh yeah, they recommended I try a chiropractor because they thought the vagus nerve might be "pinched." Although it was nice to be cracked on a regular basis, it didn't help. Next up was months of acupuncture too. I was jabbed with countless needles all over my body and left alone in a dark room three times a week. I gave it the old college try, but it didn't really help.

They even suggested a stomach pacemaker, so my vagus nerve could be triggered to tell my stomach to start digesting. I was all over the gastroparesis message boards and read about people who had stomach pacemakers, and they were much sicker than I was. While I don't like to play the "who is sicker" game at all, I thought it was best to put the pacemaker on hold until I ran out of other options.

During this entire time of second-guessing every diagnosis and moving on to the next one, the gluten-free diet was always an underlying factor. While I had been given blood tests and endoscopies (although not really done to the standards set by the Celiac Disease Foundation), they all came back relatively negative. I continued the diet because they suspected I might have an issue with some food, and they wanted

---

[10] Idiopathic meant there was no real cause, not that it was caused by idiots or only afflicted idiots. Although sometimes I feel like idiots cause my all of my problems.

my stomach to be as happy as possible while I was putting it through all of the other tests. The detective in me was losing his shit with this unsolved case.

However, it wasn't until I went to Mayo Clinic that I really understood that a positive celiac disease diagnosis could have been the cause of all of my issues all along.

As you can see, getting diagnosed took several years and several doctors. The cast and crew of my diagnosis included my general primary-care practitioner, my first gastroenterologist, a surgeon, my second gastroenterologist, and a host of additional tests done by Mayo Clinic. I mention my "cast" because it was not an easy process to get diagnosed. More than once I was even told I wasn't a celiac.

Most people would harbor incredible ill will toward their doctors for not being able to get it right—and I would understand them *completely*. There are popular blog posts with comments that could fill a room, written by people ranting about their doctors and their misdiagnoses. It really is enough to turn people against the system.

I try not to get angry toward my doctors because they did the best they could with what they knew about celiac disease and what they knew about my symptoms. But to be honest, I didn't *look* like a typical celiac—although I was a duck, I didn't look or quack like one—which led to puzzled doctors. The problem is, there are too many ducks out there that *don't quack*. The symptoms of celiac disease are so varied that if doctors apply their rules to only one set of symptoms, they can't and won't find the needle in the haystack.

I think the medical system *as a whole* needs to learn more about this multi-system, multi-symptom disease instead of assuming they should just test patients that have the runs after eating a loaf of bread.

I hear horror stories from my own readers about their diagnoses, and I want to run screaming and rip my hair out. Consistently, patients are being tested for celiac via blood work and endoscopy when they are completely gluten free (thus negating the results) or they are told to just "try it out" and eat gluten-free without *any* testing. Instead of their doctors testing them proactively, some of my readers (who have one of the many symptoms) have to beg their doctors to be tested. Then they come back to the blog and ask how long they have to eat gluten before their test. Apparently these doctors don't know the standard—even though it's easily found on places like the Celiac Disease Foundation website. And too often the ones not following the protocols are specialists, not just general family-practice doctors (although I think all doctors should know about celiac regardless).

I hate to admit it, but we're just not *there* yet with the diagnosis process. Is it because celiac disease is treated with food instead of medicine—is that what trips doctors up? Is it because not every doctor knows the ins and outs of the disease? Are they just not trained in-depth about celiac disease when they study autoimmune diseases? Do they all still suspect that it's a "rare" disease instead of one that affects more than one in 133 people? I've heard many stories about doctors and nurses who weren't trained extensively in celiac disease in school, and really only found out about it from their own experiences with the disease. It is terrifying to see what some of *you* have faced in your own quest for a diagnosis. *Terrifying.*

Because I wasn't complacent in my first, second, or even third diagnosis, I want others to take their health into their own hands with the same passion. I know that's why I stress accurate testing for those that think gluten might be a problem. Please consult someone who knows what they are doing before you give up gluten permanently or try giving up gluten for health reasons. At the same time, trust your body. If you had a celiac test that was negative, but you still get incredibly sick because of gluten, then stay off of gluten! I'm just hoping we can eventually live in a world where testing is done by educated professionals, regulated by professional medical organizations, and encouraged among the general population.

Getting Diagnosed:
The Dream Scenario That
No One Ever Gets to Have

I was far from the dream diagnosis at first. Clearly, if you just finished the last chapter, you must be thinking, "Jesus! How the hell did she end up with a celiac disease diagnosis after being first diagnosed with a trillion other issues?"

I think that's why I'm now so passionate about people getting diagnosed. I don't want them to suffer for years after a misdiagnosis or for them to have to make assumptions about their own health. Hey, if the doctors can't do it (and according to the last chapter's rants many of them can't), why can't we just do it ourselves? Take your health into your own hands. Read up on how to be properly diagnosed. Find a doctor who understands your needs and how to diagnose you and treat you.

I get questioned all the time about the right way to get diagnosed. It seems like doctors are so test-happy for celiac (or just have no batshit idea of what to actually test for or how to test for it) that they're willing to do blood tests and endoscopies on people who aren't even eating gluten. As it stands now, in order to get results from either test, you must be currently consuming gluten. That's why I can't stand it when people say that their doctors told them to just stop eating gluten to see if they feel better. That's great, but what if you feel better and still want a diagnosis? Then you're going to have to go back to feeling like shit and eating high doses of poison (a.k.a. gluten) to get your body wrecked again so you can actually have antibodies in your system for the test! That's happened to me multiple times, and I do not recommend it.

Once I got to Mayo Clinic, I started to understand a better way to go about testing. I wish I had had the foresight to visit the informative websites of the Celiac Disease Foundation and the National Foundation for Celiac Awareness when I was first thought to have an issue with gluten many moons ago. Maybe then I would have demanded to be tested the proper way for celiac disease, even if just to rule it out.

First, the process starts with a suspicion. Does your "tummy" hurt after eating? Does a bagel make you bloated? Do you have diarrhea? Constipation? An itchy rash on your extremities that you just can't stop scratching? Have you lost weight without trying lately? Have chronic fatigue? You could start with something like this, or one of the other hundreds of suspected symptoms of celiac disease.

For me, it was just that I ran out of other options.

Then, you'd go to your general practitioner or gastroenterologist and you cross your fingers and ask Oz the great and powerful wizard that you get the following tests done (in this order).

I. BLOOD TEST

This test would be done when you're still eating a full-gluten diet, or have been eating gluten for several weeks. According to their website, Celiac Disease Foundation currently recommends four weeks.

As of the time this book was published, Celiac Disease Foundation's website recommends the following tests:

+ Anti-tissue transglutaminase antibody (tTG—IgA and IgG)
+ Anti-endomysial antibody (EMA-IgA)
+ Anti-deaminated gliadin peptide (DGP—IgA and IgG)

+ Total serum IgA
+ Anti-gliadin antibody (AgA—IgG and IgA)

Feel free to show this list to your provider, because God knows I have no idea what each of these are (even with CDF's explanation online). All I know is that my blood test was borderline every time I took it, so it was of no use to me at all. However, I do encourage everyone to start with the blood test before moving forward in the process, even though I hear stories of people who had negative blood tests but still feel awful eating gluten. I recommend to those unfortunate people that they should follow through with the process (an endoscopy while eating a full-gluten diet) to rule out celiac disease before giving up on wheat forever.

2. UPPER ENDOSCOPY

Ah, the "gold standard" of celiac diagnosis—the good old endoscopy. According to some organizations like Celiac Disease Foundation, this exciting procedure typically requires you to be on a full-gluten diet for between four and six weeks before the test. However, Mayo Clinic recommended more than five weeks on a full-gluten diet for me, and I believe they go up to twelve weeks for some patients now. The upper endoscopy will confirm the diagnosis, and you can see exactly how damaged your villi are.

My biopsied villi were not that damaged at six weeks, but Mayo suspected that if I went the full twelve weeks I would probably see more damage. After my mouth melting away for five weeks, I was pretty stoked that I didn't have to do the full twelve. I don't know what would have happened after twelve weeks, but I'm pretty sure it wouldn't have been pretty. There's more about preparing for your endoscopy in a later chapter.

3. GENETIC TESTING

This is typically done if an endoscopy shows signs of damage but a blood test is negative or inconclusive (like mine), or your biopsy was performed while still eating gluten free (seriously doctors, get it together). Genetic testing is an *expensive* part of the celiac disease experience.

Lucky for me, at the time of testing, I had already met my insurance's insanely high deductible and had already spent my entire savings account at Mayo Clinic.

With a simple blood test, they can test the HLA genes—specifically DQ2 and DQ8. While your genetic test can't tell you if you have *active* celiac disease now (as it shows you only the *potential* for these genes to be turned on), the absence of these genes basically excludes celiac disease. I don't know much about the specifics of this test—probably because I'm not a genetic scientist. If I were, I would probably be Dr. Henry Wu from Jurassic Park and use my powers for evil to create a swarm of velociraptors instead of working on the celiac gene, but everyone has their own calling, I guess.

Bingo—I had the genes. I bet I also have the genes for a winning personality, but they couldn't test that at Mayo Clinic without approval from my primary-care physician.

4. EMOTIONAL SUPPORT

I wholeheartedly believe that everyone who gets a celiac disease diagnosis should have some sort of freebie punch card to see a therapist or counselor. I really believe in the power of emotional support, through support groups or by paying a professional to walk you through the emotions associated with a diagnosis of a long-term illness. There's more on the power of support later in this book, but I believe this is one of the most important parts of the process. If you've been diagnosed, don't go without support. You'll need it along your journey, just as bad as you'll need a good gluten-free cookie recipe (but don't come to me for that).

5. WORK WITH A NUTRITIONIST

I chose to work with a naturopath on my nutrition because I also wanted to undergo additional food-sensitivity testing and seek natural treatments for endometriosis. I had a recommendation for a close naturopath, and although she didn't take insurance, she sounded like a real naturopathic badass.[11] While I don't recommend a naturopath for everyone, I do recommend that you visit a nutritionist or a doctor who specializes in nutrition.

Celiac disease can rob you of important nutrients because the villi are stunted and can't absorb all the goodies from your food. I believe this is why I put on so much weight when I went from gluten full to gluten free. I'm pretty sure my body was incredibly happy that it could finally eat things. Even though my villi were not that blunted, my anemia went away on a gluten-free diet, and I finally looked healthy.

My results showed that I was low in iron, calcium, D, magnesium, B, C, CoQ10 and a handful more. I was put on numerous vitamin supplements. Again, these are things I wouldn't know if I just left the doctor's office with a diagnosis. In order to feel the best that I could, I sought out a doctor to check my nutrition and nutrient deficiencies.

Today's Dietician said in their 2012 article "Gluten Free and Healthy," that iron, folate, calcium and vitamin D are the first to go, and then the longer the disease remains untreated, additional vitamins (A, D, E and K), carbs and fats are not absorbed. See how important it is to be diagnosed, to stop eating gluten, start eating well, and get your nutrients checked?

Nutrition counseling was also very helpful after diagnosis, as I learned more about what I could eat (that was gluten free of course) in order to help naturally how I felt. I am disappointed in myself that I didn't seek help with nutrition earlier in my diagnostic process, but I need to be happy that I eventually got help. No use kicking myself in

---

[11] I could write an entire chapter (and get the associated hate mail) about my experience with naturopathic medicine. As someone so rooted in studying science and traditional medicine, the thought of tinctures, homeopathy and acupuncture reminds me more of Harry Potter-esque magic than what I considered to be "real" medicine. However, part of me really *wants* to believe that there's something real and effective there. With so many people in our community raving about naturopaths, I think there's *something* there. Is it for me? Not necessarily, but I like to have a full spectrum of help available when in need.

my own butt, because God knows I might break an osteopenia-inflicted hip or something in the process.

6. BONE DENSITY SCREENING

Speaking of bones like an eighty-year-old, apparently it is common for Mayo Clinic to follow up with bone-density screenings, since I was robbed of calcium to make my bones strong and healthy.

While my bones showed only osteopenia (lower-than-normal bone density, but too high to be considered osteoporosis), I was kind of bummed that my bones weren't made of steel. I've never broken a bone, although I have dislocated things several times. Great—I had one more thing to worry about.

After that screening, every time I fell (which happens more often than you would think for a mostly-sober person) I was petrified that I would look down and see a bone sticking out of my leg like a scene from *Shark Week*. I don't know if I can blame gluten ataxia for my clumsiness, but I'm super happy that I made it to thirty without breaking every major bone in my body.

7. FOLLOW UP CARE

After I was officially diagnosed, I had a whole year to be as gluten free as I could before my follow-up endoscopy and blood work. Mayo Clinic wanted to make sure that I was healing appropriately and that all of the markers that flared up when I binged on gluten were gone after a year. Only after you receive follow-up care after your initial diagnosis can you finally feel like you're on the right path to healing with this disease.

It's my hope that everyone monitors their own health as much as I did in the years following my diagnosis. I take celiac disease very seriously, and you should too if you've been diagnosed. There's more evidence out there that proves the importance of a strict gluten-free diet. As I wrote this book, a study came out that showed increased lymphoma risk for celiacs who have ongoing intestinal damage. Yeah, scary stuff, but that type of research helps validate the fact that we need to take this seriously.

Please note that even though I talk a lot about celiac disease and the diagnosis process, that doesn't mean that I don't have mad love for you even if you don't have the same genes as me. If you went through the testing process and it turns out you *don't* have an autoimmune disease—congratulations! I know many people with *non-celiac gluten sensitivity* (NCGS) who are much more sensitive to gluten than I am, so I share the love with the non-celiac segment when I talk about living life gluten free. If we all eat in the same buffet line at conferences, you *know* I still love you. Unless you bought this book because you read *Wheat Belly* and you think I'm going to give you diet tips. Stop eating our food at conferences, please.

Once Mayo Clinic took me on, I went through all the rigors of testing again to go through *their* process and procedures. I again had a lukewarm blood test, but my genetic testing was positive. Like Shakira said, hips don't lie—and genes don't either. It was a relief to know that I'm susceptible to celiac because knowing me, my genes would have been triggered eventually even if my biopsy didn't show I had it. My genetics always give me the *best* things, like curly hair that will turn into a serious fro should it not be controlled with serum.

After my endoscopy and my final diagnosis, I was sent on my way with some Mayo-branded literature (albeit from 2009), some photocopies of book excerpts, and a packet from the US Department of Health and Human services. I was impressed, as this was way more than the other doctors provided. For what other disease do you get the answer "just Google it," as a game plan?

Like most of the information in this book, I wish I knew then what I know now. Again, if you think your doctor has no idea what they're doing when it comes to testing for celiac—then run. RUN. Seek a doctor who has pride in their knowledge of celiac disease or NCGS. I promise you, they are out there. You may have to drive to the next town, or the town after that, but it will be worth it for your health.

Returning to Gluten:
The Gluten Challenge and
Reuniting With Wheat

People ask me why I decided to get "tested" for celiac disease when I was already eating gluten free, knowing full well I would have to go back on a gluten-full diet.[12] There are a few reasons why I decided to get back together with gluten for the gluten challenge[13].

1. **I needed to know because I didn't have the typical symptoms.** Maybe it was something else? As described in the previous chapters, no one had any idea what it was: food sensitivities, faulty gallbladder, broken vagus nerve, IBS, arthritis, anxiety, spasmodic intestines, ulcer, GERD, etc. I needed a definitive answer—what was my problem? I think if I had all of the typical

---

[12] I use quotes on "tested" only because I was supposedly tested several times before going gluten free seriously, so *this* test was like the super-serious official test. This test was like the SATs of celiac, and the other tests were like my prep courses that I apparently failed.

[13] The "gluten challenge" is the commonly referenced term of going back on a full gluten-containing diet before undergoing tests for celiac disease. This generally entails 4–12 weeks of eating several servings of gluten daily.

symptoms of a celiac, and reacted poorly (and/or crapped my pants) upon eating gluten, then I might have just removed it from my diet and been happy. But that wasn't my story. I needed to know an answer. *Any answer.*

2. **Since I didn't have "traditional" symptoms, I knew that I could survive without the day-by-day symptoms that disable most celiacs during testing.** I approached eating gluten again with excitement. Although I was super grossed out knowing that my insides were going to hell, it was still pretty awesome to walk through the grocery aisles and pull anything I wanted into my cart. I just wanted to spin around and sing like a Disney princess in the middle of my grocery store. "Ohhhhhhhh, isn't this ah-ma-zing! I can eat anything I want! I don't even have to read a laaaaaaaaaaaaaaaaaabel!" It was great, until weird things happened, but whatever. I was still excited to eat my Trader Joe's Cinnamon Swirl bread by the bag-full.

3. **I wanted an official diagnosis because that doesn't make me a hypochondriac.** I often told my mother, "I'm not a hypochondriac if every time I go to the doctor, I am diagnosed with something new." It seemed with every doctor appointment I'd have more symptoms and another random diagnosis that they were stuck trying to figure out or piece together. If I didn't have a diagnosis, I didn't think that people would take me seriously. I didn't think that my employer would let me take so many sick days. I didn't think I could be happy until I had a label. While most people fight to reject the labels that are forced upon them by society, I was desperately seeking mine out so I could know I wasn't loony.

So many people ask me for advice about whether or not they should get tested or just go gluten free and see if they feel better. I ask them these important follow-up questions.

If you go gluten free and you feel better, would you be willing to give up gluten for the rest of your life—to never, ever cheat on it again, even if it is just a crumb? Are you committed to asking about cross-contamination procedures at every restaurant you ever visit? Are you okay with throwing out all of your current kitchen equipment (including wooden utensils and your toaster) and replacing it all?

Because if you *don't know* if you are celiac or not—*assume the worst.* If you refuse to get tested, you will never know if you have celiac disease or non-celiac gluten sensitivity. While they may act the same, they are *very* different.

With celiac disease, a speck or a small crumb of gluten can cause serious damage, especially if you "cheat" and have "just a little gluten" because you feel better when removing *most* gluten. Even if you feel better gluten free, you have to be *so much more careful* than just ordering off the gluten-free menu at any restaurant you patronize.

Are you willing to undergo more tests for other autoimmune diseases? Are you willing to get your bones scanned to measure bone density? Are you willing to check your nutrient levels and continue to visit a nutritionist until you are fully healed? These are all things that should be done when assuming that you are a celiac.

I think that the above is one of my biggest issues with gluten-free living as a trend: People are going GF without realizing the repercussions of going undiagnosed. Sure, you may *feel* better, but if you're a celiac, more needs to be done to keep your body safe and healthy. If you go undiagnosed, you may not do any of the things you need to do to really get well.

And *then* when these people actually want to get diagnosed (maybe because they had a story like mine or maybe they just wanted to save money on their taxes), they have to go *back* on gluten in order to get positive results on the "gold standard" biopsy. This is a difficult thing to tell people, especially if they feel so much better *off* of gluten. It's better to get everything taken care of while you are still eating gluten—I promise.

At first, going back to gluten (for the sake of science, *obviously*) was easy. After numerous Disney-esque moments twirling through the aisles of grocery stores not reading any labels, I got used to eating gluten-full food. I could visit all my favorite restaurants and have all of my favorite menu items I had been craving. I could buy all of those grocery items that I was used to scoffing at as I wheeled my cart feverishly by previously.

The following list includes the items that I went absolute apeshit over during my gluten binge:

1. Everything Bagels. I don't know how Einstein Bagels does it, but their everything bagel is a magical experience. It's chewy, it toasts amazingly, and has the best blend of spices to create that perfect "Everything" experience. This cannot be replicated in gluten-free form—believe me, I've tried every "everything bagel" in GF form. I want to weep when I taste the gluten-free version, as it can't live up to what I remember.

2. Subway sandwiches. Yes, their meat is a bit slimy and over-processed. Their vegetables are sub-par imitations of what should be in a real sandwich. But their bread—OMG their bread. There are like a million varieties of it, and it always smells so damn good! And you can see it baking in their little clear square ovens. It's magic. I don't miss their sandwich fillings, but I would totally eat a Subway sandwich every day just so I could have that bread. If you've ever ordered a salad at Subway after being diagnosed, you will understand my disappointment. I still can't walk into a Subway, but if they launch their gluten-free bread nationwide, I might change my mind.

3. Olive Garden. Don't judge me, but man, did Olive Garden know how to cook up some pasta. They had this amazing shrimp scampi that was so oily and garlicky and so perfect. There's no way I could replicate it—possibly because I'm just really terrible in the kitchen. However, when I had it during the binge, it was significantly less amazing than I remembered it

to be. The pasta tasted overly sticky and doughy (could it have been all the gluten?).

4. Wendy's breaded chicken sandwiches. One of the first items I ate was the crispy chicken sandwich. Not only was I getting gluten with their tasty, soft buns, but also with their breaded chicken breasts. I can't even tell you about the experience of eating one of these for the first time. It was so private, I wrote about it in my journal and then hugged the paper drive-thru bag as I fell asleep.

5. McDonald's wraps. There is no way to explain why I like these wraps. Looking at it, it's a poorly constructed wrap on a bland flour tortilla with an over-seasoned piece of chicken breast, occasional lettuce, and a honey mustard or ranch sauce. But, when that warm chicken torpedo enters your mouth, it's just delicious.

6. Those sugar cookies with the pink frosting that are approximately one thousand calories per bite at the grocery store in the bakery section. I don't know what they're called, but I'm pretty sure I've called them "Satan's cookies" before. I don't know what they're made of either, but I'm pretty sure it's a recipe that Paula Deen would be proud of.

7. Cinnamon swirl bread from Trader Joe's. This has to be the best thing that Trader Joe's has ever made (besides the gluten-free Jo-Jo's a.k.a. Oreos that they recently launched). Imagine soft whole-wheat bread with cinnamon and sugar swirled into the bread itself. This bread is perfect. Or should I say, it was perfect until I had to choke down three slices of this a day. It got old quick.

8. Paradise Bakery cookies. I still wipe away a little tear when I pass by one of these in the mall or in the airport (especially when I'm *hangry* waiting for a delayed flight). Their chocolate chip nut cookie is one of the best things in the universe. It achieves a texture and mouth feel that is not replicable in my kitchen,

even with all the butter in the world. And the smell—that smell! You can't escape the smell of those cookies, even when you walk by the store in an outdoor mall. The cookie smell can penetrate through concrete walls.

I had six weeks, yes SIX whole weeks of eating gluten. So while I was going crazy my body was going Captain Insano on me. I ended up feeling like crap—just some general malaise, anxiety, etc. However, I was pretty excited that I wasn't dying. I thought *maybe* I could go back to gluten and nothing really bad would happen. Maybe I was just a *little* celiac? I should have known that being a little celiac is like being a little pregnant. You either are, *or you're not.*

One night my shoulder started itching like crazy. Upon inspecting my shoulder and its nonstop itching at dinner (because I'm classy), I found two clusters of bumps. I thought they were spider bites. I don't know when, where, or how I would be exposed to such a mean spider, but I just made assumptions. When those itchy bumps didn't go away for a while, I went to the MinuteClinic at CVS. I don't really know what they could have done if they were spider bites, but like most things that go wrong with my body, I just wanted a professional to assure me that I wasn't dying. They thought it was just dermatitis from something—even though I didn't have anything new that would trigger it (e.g., new bra, new purse, new pet—unless you count a new boyfriend). I put steroid cream on it for a few days. I kept eating gluten, and I kept being an emotional beast.

While high on gluten, I made terrible mistakes. These mistakes included sobbing at a ticket booth to a poor woman who misplaced my "will call" tickets for an outdoor music festival. It also included mistakenly making out with a dude who was definitely not my type (although he recently became religious, so I have high hopes for his new life in the church without me). I don't want to blame gluten for my life's *faux pas*, but I will anyway.

In an odd turn of events, I went to the dermatologist soon after for my annual skin cancer check-up and inquired about the rash. She inspected it and took my history with it. And she simply said, "Sounds like shingles." I'm sorry, what? *Shingles*? You mean the thing that old people get and have in those TV commercials? No, *not* cool. So, because it was a derivative of the Herpes/chicken pox virus, I had to take Valtrex for weeks just in case it was shingles. I was worried that I would have to call the dude and say, "Hey, I hope I didn't give you shingles—just in case you have a compromised immune system like I do. Good luck with Jesus!"

When my five weeks with gluten were done, I told my gastroenterologist at Mayo about the rash drama, and she said, "It was probably dermatitis herpetiformis[14]." Duh. I guess we'll never know what the mysterious rash was, and I guess I won't care (other than thinking the "shingles vaccine" sign at my grocery store is specifically talking to me every time I see it). Knowing what I know now, I probably wouldn't have panicked and instead would have just called the gastro to get anti-itch medication for what probably was DH, but what's the fun in knowing it all? It's fun to go bat-shit crazy your first go-round, *right*?

---

[14] According to the National Foundation for Celiac Awareness, "Dermatitis Herpetiformis (DH) is a severe, itchy, blistering skin manifestation of celiac disease that is genetically determined and is not contagious." While not all celiacs have DH, I've had many afflicted celiacs tell me it's not very fun. If you've got a weird rash, get that bad boy checked out!

Does My Villi
Look Fat in That Picture?
A Tale of Upper Endoscopies

Before my Mayo Clinic endoscopy, I had two with another doctor. Unfortunately I was not eating enough gluten long enough to show positive results. While I could be angry about having to undergo procedures that basically proved nothing, at least I got some good sympathy comments on Facebook. Hopefully, by taking the right steps to assure your tests are accurate, you can limit unnecessary endoscopies for your diagnosis story.

Endoscopies are really nothing to be worried about, so put the bottle of Xanax down. Basically all you have to do is stop eating the midnight before the endoscopy—because no one wants to see a half-digested Egg McMuffin in your stomach during the procedure. Pray that you have an early start time at the hospital so you don't die of starvation before you go under. Being hungry in a hospital gown hooked up to an IV is the worst—I've done it way too many times.

A pre-op nurse once told me that you don't want to go under when you're cranky and bitchy. Then again, I *may* have told the surgery staff that

I wasn't very good under anesthesia and that I am likely to get mouthy at the staff.[15] The wise Yoda pre-op nurse said that whatever mood you are in when you go under sedation is the mood that your body is in when it goes into surgery. So, in order to have a positive surgery and a positive recovery, you had to go into sedation happy. Personally, I think that could all be the biggest crock of bullshit ever, spoon-fed to assholes like me who hate surgery and hate late surgeries even more. But, in every surgery after that one, I really tried to go into sedation on a positive note. Or just ask for enough Xanax in my IV to feign happiness.

An endoscopy is typically a quick procedure, which is great news. You'll get sedated enough for you to go to la-la twilight land, and then they insert a tube with a camera down your throat and start taking pictures when they enter your stomach and then throughout your small intestine. After they are done snapping some glamour shots of your insides, they take a couple of samples of your small intestine in a few spots so they can check out your villi and what's going on with your cells down there. Don't worry; you won't feel anything. Plus, your villi have probably been through enough with celiac disease that I wouldn't worry about their hurt feelings if they weren't selected for the biopsy.

You'll wake up all foggy and magical, and the doctor will talk to you and whomever you bring along to drive you home. Then about an hour later you'll actually wake up (meaning you'll be coherent) and ask where you are, how you got dressed, and what happened during the procedure. If your helper person has never picked up anyone from surgery, he or she will probably wonder if you had a lobotomy while you were under, but it's just the lovely side effects of anesthesia. You won't remember a damn thing. In fact, *it's kind of funny.*

However, now is where I have to give you a very real, very important warning. Before you go under sedation, give your VIP helper your phone. Tell them exactly what I'm telling you right now. Say:

---

[15] I just remember yelling at a recovery nurse after my first surgery, "Why don't YOU put my f-ing pants on!" I should probably find that nurse and bake her some cupcakes or something as a belated apology.

"While I may look and sound like I am awake and highly function-ing when I wake up, I am not. While I may dress myself and ask the doctor questions, I am not really functioning. When I ask for my phone and I tell you, 'It's okay, I'm awake,' I am not. Do NOT give me my phone until several hours after I first come to after surgery. Perhaps let me have a little nap first. Let me eat a few gluten-free saltine crackers and have some ginger ale. Let me watch at least one episode of my favorite TV show on Netflix. Regardless, do NOT give me my phone until you are sure that I am awake, can remember things, and make good judgments."

I sound serious *because I am serious.*

Here are some dangerous things I have done while my mom/boyfriend thought I was "awake" from anesthesia, but I wasn't:

+ Posted status updates on Facebook about what my doctor found inside my stomach, inside my abdominal cavity, and inside my rectum. I shit you not. Every time, my mom gives me my phone and I think it's incredibly appropriate to tell all of my friends that, surprisingly to my doctor, my ovaries look perfect. Maybe you're really close, honest, and "real" with your Facebook friends. However, you might want to think before you post about any of your internal organs on a public or semi-public domain. All of my Facebook friends—luckily—are used to it.

+ Posted Instagram photos of myself under deep sedation. Now, I'm very against posting anything on Instagram where I am not wearing a bra. It doesn't even have to be a photo of my torso. Just posting a picture of my face where I am not wear-ing a bra—I just feel like people will *know*. So, needless to say, photos of me without make-up in a hospital gown without a bra giving a thumbs-up with the oxygen tubes still in my nose was not what I really wanted to post. However, under the magical fairy dust of post-surgery, I thought it would be a perfect shot. Hours after surgery, when I am safe at home, eating food and recovering from the surgery, I scroll through my Instagram and yell, "Dammit Mom!" She falls for it every surgery.

✦ But my favorite has to be the e-mail—yes e-mail—that I sent to a boy that I wasn't even *really* dating: it was basically a break-up e-mail. I'm pretty sure it went something like, "Oh? How am I doing? I just got back from surgery. I'm in pain. THANKS FOR ASKING." It probably ended with something dramatic. Maybe it didn't even end at all. Maybe I just pressed "send." Regardless, that was the last time I talked to him. Probably for the best, right?

After your endoscopy, you should have a follow-up appointment (or at least a phone call) with the doctor to go over your results. For me, this phone call seemed to take forever to receive, like the world stopped and wanted me to just sit and panic over the question of "to be or not to be a celiac." Of course, my phone call *did indeed* confirm active celiac disease—which kind of wasn't a surprise after my genetic-testing results. At least my genes were being active, even if I just wanted to stay home on the couch.

Let's Talk About Butts:
A Story of a Girl, Her Rectum,
and the Scope That Loved Her

I take some odd sort of pride in the fact that I had a colonoscopy before I was thirty years old. But, I kind of wish I did it before my parents did so I could rub the fact that they are terrible whiners in their face. I remember them telling me horror stories about spending an entire day in the bathroom, and it mortified me. No one wants to think about their parents pooping their brains out. Or "making love"—*either/or*. It was such a disturbing story to me that when I was forced to have my first colonoscopy when I was twenty-nine, I panicked.

I spent hours on the Internet learning all about what happens during the colonoscopy prep. The actual procedure didn't scare me, but I was totally scared that I would poop my pants during this prep time. I've had the occasional bouts of diarrhea, but it's not really part of my regular life (please don't hate me, "traditional" celiacs!). Laxatives were never really my bag. I never took a laxative that wasn't prescribed by my doctor (and that was just a few doses of MiraLAX to help the train to get to the station on time). I've really regulated what I eat to *avoid* "the squirts" from sketchy food, so the thought of seeking that out just seemed a little wrong.

My amazing boyfriend (commonly referenced as Non-GFBF—more on him later), told me that he was going to be out of town when my colonoscopy was scheduled. He'd be in Vegas nonetheless—what an asshole. Part of me was sad that I didn't have anyone to hold my hand while I was going through it, but part of me was really happy that I was going to have the whole house in which to mope about. And if—just if—for some reason I sharted on the couch, I could easily clean it up by the time he got home. That way there wouldn't have to be some deep dark poop secret shared between us. Not that I wouldn't consider that a real "bonding" moment in our relationship, but I'd rather let our love grow without it.

I opted for the most expensive prep—MoviPrep, which did *not* mean that it was any tastier or any less laxative-y than the other preps—I just wanted to feel *fancy*. Fancy shits. The truth is that this prep is about fifty percent less liquid than the other preps, which for someone with gastroparesis who has a hard time drinking lots of liquid at one time, was a blessing. I visited MoviPrep's website[16] and watched all of their tutorial videos detailing the experience. The more prepared I was for this event, the less my anxiety made me want to crawl up the wall. Side note, one of MoviPrep's mantras is "strive for a clean colon," and for some reason it makes me laugh, like it belongs on some sort of motivational poster with a illustration of Rosie the Riveter or a humpback whale jumping out of the water.

I went to the store and purchased bottles of coconut water and Gatorade like I was stocking up for the apocalypse (that was about to happen in my colon). A few days before the prep you're supposed to start a low-residue diet, which is something I was familiar with from my gastroparesis days. I had to do away with high-fiber foods like raw

---

[16] Kudos for the amazing and helpful website, MoviPrep people. I'd love for you to contact me to run ads on my site. I have no shame.

fruits and veggies and whole grains. I ate a lot of pasta and cooked veggies without skin and did some juicing. I hated it because it reminded me of my days where I had to eat like that. A day before the procedure, you must go on a liquid diet. There is absolutely no advice that I can give you for this part because I abhor liquid diets. If liquid diets were a person, they'd be that girl in high school with the perfect hair and early-developing boobs who, with just one look in the lunch line, could be so cruel to you. I want to punch liquid diets in the face. Just get through it, and know that soon it will get much, *much* worse.

My first prep was set for 10 p.m. because I was assigned the split dosage (one dose the night before the procedure and one dose the day of the procedure—roughly five hours before). Why is the split-dosage prep designed to be administered so late? I don't know, but it's probably to punish you for something bad you did as a kid. As if having a colonoscopy didn't suck enough, you have to go without sleep the entire night before *while* crapping your pants. Apparently having a split dosage actually improves your chances of seeing everything during the procedure, so it's one of those things where you keep telling yourself over and over again, "It's for my health."

The videos were pretty detailed about mixing the solution they provided. "Pour A into the bottle of warm water, and then pour B into the bottle. Shake until it looks absolutely disgusting." Or something like that. I was so hesitant about taking my first sip because I had heard how vile the liquid was. But away I went on my trip down the rabbit hole.

My bathroom was all set up for the event. I had my robe in case it got cold in the bathroom or my body was too dehydrated to produce heat. I brought a nightstand in and hooked up my MacBook. I logged into Netflix and brought in a few books just in case I got sick.

I finally took the first dose. I don't know what I expected, but I prepared myself for the worst. I was actually pleasantly surprised at the taste. It tasted like lemonade but a little chalky. I drank the first eight ounces and set my timer for fifteen minutes to prepare for the second dose.

When I look back now, I guess I didn't think about the science behind the laxative before I started my prep. Clearly, the liquid laxative needed time to get through my system before it started working. However, I sat on the toilet immediately, expecting a full system blow-out within the first few minutes. Nothing happened except my butt got numb from sitting, wishing, waiting on the hard, cold plastic seat. At that point, I wished I had invested in one of those old-people cushioned toilet seats. I decided it was safe to venture into the living room and walk around a bit.

I took my second and third doses. *Still nothing.* By now the "pleasantly surprising" taste I mentioned earlier had morphed into the most disgusting fake-lemon-like grimy liquid that I could think of. It started to remind me of a really disgusting *faux* lemon scent. Recently, a reader said he was nauseated after his wife brought home dishwashing detergent because it reminded him of the prep.[17] Soon I was well on my way to the rinse cycle.

I started getting all crampy and super uncomfortable, like how I imagine those pregnant girls are in the delivery room on *16 and Pregnant* (I watch a lot of daytime TV reruns). I walked around the living room a bit more, hoping that I wouldn't have to resort to doing a round of P90X in order to dislodge my dinner from a week ago. Sitting on the toilet seemed like the only reasonable thing to do, since I just got so bored of waiting. I prayed that something would happen so I could *get the show on the road*. At that point, I started panicking that I hadn't done it right. What if nothing happens? Would I have to reschedule and do this all again?! As I took my last dose, I started to feel very nauseated because I was so full of this terrible poop juice. As someone with a genuine fear of vomiting, this didn't help my panic. I'm pretty sure this wasn't the first time I sat on the toilet and cried, *and I'm pretty sure it won't be the last*.

Once the *magic* started, I was actually relieved. It meant that I wasn't doing it wrong and that I didn't have to repeat the procedure. And to

---

[17] He totally nailed it; the prep tasted like what powdered lemon Cascade probably tastes like (without the whole dishwashing my insides action . . . but kind of still like dishwashing my insides).

me, that meant that I wouldn't have to throw it all up and thus throw it all away. My demeanor was shockingly different after I felt this relief. And let me get real with you here—*I started laughing.*

Farting, by nature, is hilarious to me. I've never met a fart I couldn't laugh about. And although I'd never be so lax as to have flatulence in public for giggles (Non-GFBF will call my bluff on this one in the editing process, I'm sure), I find it funny when it happens at inopportune moments. So when the farts started, I couldn't stop myself from laughing. Like, schoolgirl laughter. Like the kind of laughter that happens and you can't stop and then your side hurts—that laughter. The cats came into the bathroom and got genuinely scared of the noises, which of course, made me laugh even more. After the farts, came the *real* experience.

The only true way to describe what happens to you while getting prepped for a colonoscopy is like going number one out of your number two. I've (luckily) never had the experience outside of a colonoscopy. It just doesn't stop. It. Doesn't. Stop. I've had horrific food poisoning before. It was the kind of awful food poisoning where you had to make the no-win choice of vomiting on yourself or pooping your pants.[18] While I'd much rather have a colonoscopy (at least with that you can prepare and catch up on some Netflix), it's about the same sense of urgency that's hard to replicate outside of eating bad Greek food.

But listen, you just *have* to buckle down and do it. Everyone has to have a colonoscopy eventually. There are no ifs, ands, or butts (seriously butts) about it. If you're lucky, you won't have to have it until you're fifty. If you're unlucky, you'll have one earlier than that. But, you've just got to grin and bear it. Think of it like your personal version of the Master Cleanse you never wanted to go through—but much quicker. Hopefully you'll find it a funny (or briefly entertaining) experience like I did.

---

[18] Our entire office was once served a steaming platter of feces at a luncheon. I mean, it definitely felt like we ate that, because more than half of the office was violently ill the following days. I mean, like hospital ill. I never wanted my mother so badly as the days I was stuck in the bathroom, praying it would all end. I wish someone would invent an emergency food poisoning kit with collapsible bucket for instances like these.

Here are some suggestions for surviving the prep:

1. **Stock up on liquid that tastes good.** This includes coconut water, Gatorade, sparkling water, etc. I really liked chicken broth because it made me feel like I was eating something wholesome instead of just chugging water. Plus, the hot liquid was a change from the cold Gatorade. Just make sure that you get gluten-free chicken broth. Don't get glutened while your guard is down! Any liquid you drink has to be close to clear. Dark-colored beverages like red or purple liquid (e.g., cranberry juice or grape juice) could skew the results, and trust me, you want to avoid going through this twice because you mistakenly bought the wrong-colored liquid. Pulp is also not okay, so avoid juices that contain pulp. Avoid dairy, which wasn't a problem for me and probably won't be for you if you imagine drinking milk with what's happening inside your colon. While you can have coffee on the prep, I didn't need anything that kept me awake or kept me more "regular" than I already was.

2. **Pretend like you're at a frat party.** Chase the laxative with Gatorade and just chug it. Hold your nose if you have to. Just get it down. Imagine a crowd of drunken guys cheering you on if you have to. Drink it with a straw so you won't taste it when it goes down. Put on your old Soffe shorts with your college logo on 'em if you have to. Pound it, son!

3. **Don't be a pansy.** I know it sucks. But, again, you just have to do it. Don't cheat on your doses; follow the instructions to a "T." Fast when you are supposed to fast according to your doctor. Don't cheat and have a Larabar. Trust me, it will suck *so* much more to have to redo the prep because you did it wrong. Trust me, I'm a pansy.

The actual colonoscopy procedure was less exciting (*thank God*) than the prep. However—in true Erica fashion—I did have a bit of a scare when I checked into Mayo Clinic. They asked me the last time I had solid food, and I told them that I ate lunch about six hours before the prep process started—technically the day before the prep. The check-in ladies said that I would have to do my whole colonoscopy over again. I stared at them in disbelief and informed them that I was called by a nurse at Mayo and given instructions that I could eat up until several hours before I started the prep the night before (my first split dosage was 10 p.m.). The staff was adamant. I would have to repeat the cleanse; my body just wasn't "empty" enough to see inside there. When I was told that, I felt a mixture of vomiting, crying, and screaming (also, kind of like I had to poop again, but I think that was just the prep talking). I had just dumped everything out of my system in the most nonpolite way possible and starved myself, and they wanted me to do this *again*? No thank you. I demanded they put the scope up my butt that instant, and swore how clean my bowel movements were. I had never fought so hard to convince someone that I had done an excellent job of defecating.

Luckily, they did follow through with my scope, and I pestered them about giving better prep information to those with split-dosage night prep instead of the day-before prep. It's confusing enough as it is to know *what* to drink and *when*, but way more confusing if you get mixed messages on when you have to stop eating.

I was put under and didn't remember a thing until I was home (see previous snippet about anesthesia and endoscopies). When I finally came to, my mom got to show me all the pictures from inside my rectum— obviously my favorite part of the day! Luckily, Mayo didn't have any polyps to take out, but they did show signs of endometriosis-like cells inside the bowel. Awesome.

If there was a Hallmark card that read "Good luck on your upcoming anal probing," I would have packaged it with your book order. Until then, I can only wish you clean and healthy insides.

Mourning the Death of Gluten: Rebirthing Your New Life Sans Gluten

Anyone who tells you that it was easy to flip the gluten-to-gluten-free switch the second they walked out of their doctor's office needs to go back and get their head examined. Much like anything pretty awful in life, getting diagnosed with a lifelong autoimmune disease requires grieving. You've got to take some time to mourn. Mourn the death of gluten, mourn the lack of choices you have in the grocery store or restaurant, mourn your old social life that included eating food with friends, and mourn the loss of your favorite snacks. Yes, that means sitting and thinking about a life without Little Debbie Snack Cakes. I know that seems like something you'd never do with tears streaming down your face, but things change when gluten is taken away from you. These feelings are all normal, I promise.

If you've just been diagnosed, you've got to take some time and be sad. Let's examine the Kübler-Ross model, also known as the five stages of grief. While this model is most often used when a person is diagnosed with a critical illness or facing the death of a loved one (pretty heavy stuff compared to the death of Little Debbie and her delicious snack cakes), it applies just as much to being diagnosed with a lifelong condition (like celiac disease).

By knowing what you'll likely face, you'll better understand what's in front of you. And if you've been diagnosed for a while like I have, you'll better understand the feelings of newbies and maybe even help them along in their recovery journey.

DENIAL

Denial is the stage where you pretend like the diagnosis didn't happen to you. Hey, maybe they just mixed up the test results, right? This is your brain's line of defense against the truth. I learned a great deal about denial when I watched the movie *He's Just Not That Into You*. And while that film (and book) focused on being in denial about the person you're dating being a total loser who hates you, it taught me some good lessons about accepting the truth that is staring you in the face.[19]

Oddly enough, because of my high-functioning villi, I've been told a few times that I did *not* have celiac disease. The first occasion was when I was not eating gluten and the doctor still ran tests (epic fail on the doctor's end). I still have the notes that said I didn't have celiac—scribbled on a piece of paper—next to the names of four new medications to help solve whatever was wrong with me that apparently wasn't this disease.

I also found a Facebook post from Thanksgiving of 2010. "Just started my day with a Starbucks breakfast sandwich, so I'm *thankful* I'm not a celiac." Ha-ha, the joke is on *you*, past Erica—because you are!

My second opportunity for easy denial came from another doctor's office. After genetic testing, one of their nurses left a message and said that I didn't have celiac—but when their office called me back a

---

[19] It also taught me that almost everyone I have ever dated was definitely not that into me—*but that's another book.*

little while later, they said that I did. I feel like my genes had a case of multiple-personality disorder.

It's easy to be in denial with so many varied symptoms of celiac, and even harder if you are one of the numerous silent/asymptomatic celiacs out there. It's probably difficult to believe that you're causing lifelong damage to your system if you don't feel a thing. While celiac makes it easy to be in denial, you can't deny that you need a lifelong strict lifestyle change upon diagnosis. It's just not fair to your body, and you can't expect your mind to heal and overcome this hurdle either.

Since I had dabbled with the game of "do I/don't I," I had always thought that when someone really got their act together and tested me for realsies, I wouldn't have celiac. I was sure that it was just a wacky gallbladder or something that could be remedied easily with surgery or controlled with a pill.

I battled with denial for a while and through several doctors. But, while denial felt so good, it also really sucked because I still had no idea what was wrong with me unless it was this all-encompassing autoimmune disease.

ANGER

This is the really fun stage where you're angry all the time (and also the stage where I wholeheartedly believe that Xanax should be handed out to any newly diagnosed person). You've realized that you really are going to have to eat gluten free for the rest of your life. There's no denying it any longer: You are sick, and you need to change your diet immediately.

You'll scream, you'll cry, you'll ask, "Why me?!?!" when you're lying in bed at night. You'll whine around the house (or in the grocery aisles) and scream, "It's not fair!" and stomp your feet like a toddler throwing a tantrum. You'll probably swear more in this stage than you ever have before.

To cope with this stage, my suggestion is to totally vent it all out. Write angry tear-stained letters to whole-wheat pasta, Dunkin' Donuts, and every other item you're so bummed about. Tell them that you will miss them dearly and you'll think about them every night.[20] Sit in your bathroom, light a candle and cry it out over the fact that you have an autoimmune disease. Shed a tear every time you hear your friends talking about staying in and ordering a pizza, and then tell them you hate them and you never want to see them again (well, never see them again as long as they're talking about pizza). Cuss out your gluten-filled food as you throw it all away in a massive trash bag. There's nothing quite as enjoyable as screaming "SCREW YOU, WHEAT THINS," as you pitch them in the trash.

And what about your parents? Oh boy, isn't genetics fun, folks? If you have celiac, someone had to give you those genes. Are you angry with your mom yet? Or maybe it was your dad? Grandma? I'm pretty sure all of this genetic talk and the awful Punnett square of genetics they handed down to me guilted my parents into buying me a car. But seriously, you can be angry at a donut, *but don't be angry with your parents*, especially if they took care of you and were incredibly supportive while you were sick (like mine). I promise they didn't give you those genes as punishment for totaling their car when you were a teenager. Although my parents *might* be the exception to that rule. Now, if your parents are *real jerks* about the whole thing, I give you every right to be angry with them and their genes.

But really, no one in your family asked for those genes. And I know you didn't either. It's *just science*. It's just how the gluten-free cookie crumbles.

BARGAINING

When it comes to being gluten free, I think that the bargaining stage is where I cheated the most. This stage is where we try to delay the

---

[20] My letter would probably sound a little like this: "Dear pink strawberry frosted Dunkin' Donut with all of your delicious sprinkles on top (heavy sobs), I HATE YOU. Why do you have to be so delicious? Why do you have to be made with refined white flour? WHY YOU? WHY ME? I never thought I'd tell you this, but I have to let you go. You can't continue to hurt me anymore!"

inevitable, or try to cope with it by delaying it or taking a less-inevitable view of it. Maybe the disease will go away if we just change our behaviors a little? Maybe if I just cut back, I'll get better? I don't have to go 100% gluten free, do I? At this point, you may try every diet under the sun to try to feel better. It has to be anything but gluten, right?

We think that the situation may change. Well—*too bad*. This isn't like some ex-boyfriend who you can beg to take you back because you promise that you can change (FYI, don't ever do this either). Being diagnosed is permanent until they find a cure—and you shouldn't hold your breath for that.

Granted, at this point in my grieving process, I didn't really know how harmful cheating (or should I say just *avoiding* gluten) was, but I swiftly learned that I wasn't getting any better by dwelling on this stage. I was not the woman I am today. I was still in love with gluten. I would order regular meals and take the bread off. I know this sounds weird, but sometimes I would eat gluten—chew it up to get the taste and texture in my mouth, and spit it up in a napkin before I could accidentally swallow it. I never asked about cross-contamination outside of the house—partly because I didn't really know it existed and partly because I didn't really *want* to know it existed. I figured, "Hey, this isn't so bad," and I figured I could live my life like that. Nope. I was still getting sick and still wasn't feeling any better.

Snap back to reality and realize that there's nothing you can do right now to change this issue that you were born with.

DEPRESSION

This is the stage where you just want to stay in bed all day and cry about it. You're not really angry anymore, just sullen and aloof, like an "emo" teenager from a Stephenie Meyer vampire book. You've now broken all of your dinnerware and have gotten out your aggression by yelling at a box of Ramen you found hiding in the back of your cupboard. So, now you're eating nothing but gluten-free cupcakes off of Chinet paper plates because you're *also* eating your feelings.

Some people just stop at this stage, and it alarms me how long they actually stay in it. Especially now that we have a ton of gluten-free packaged products out there that are so similar to what we're used to eating. Restaurants (even huge chains) have gluten-free menus. Although they're not always doing GF right, it's a sign of huge progress. Imagine being diagnosed ten, twenty, or fifty years ago. How can you be depressed knowing we have it so much better than the banana babies in the 1940s? Not that dwelling on the past is the best way to cure Debbie Downer-ism, but you can't be mad when even Betty Crocker has a cheap gluten-free cookie mix.

We've come a long way, baby.

ACCEPTANCE

Okay, are you done yet? Have you made amends to everyone you punched in the face during your anger stage? Have you thanked your boyfriend for bringing you Sprinkles GF cupcakes while you lay in bed feeling sorry for yourself? Have you changed out of those sweatpants yet?[21]

After you're done feeling sorry for yourself, buck up and realize that everything is going to be okay. Your life won't be worse; your life will only be *different*. You're going to start paying attention to everything you consume, and honestly I am happy about it now (even though it took me several years). You will start being more in tune with your body than ever before and understand the fuel it needs to run properly. And really, that letter you wrote to the pink frosted donut will seem silly a year from now.

So what comes after all the stages of grief? I'm not sure what to tell you, but it's a lifetime of being gluten free. I know that seems really overwhelming, even for someone who has done it for so long. The words "lifetime" and "forever"— those words are scary. No one likes to be just one thing forever. People constantly change. However, the one

---

[21] No judgment implied, as most of this book was written in sweat pants or yoga pants.

change that you'll never have again is a life with gluten. Like I said in the beginning, it does get easier. You adjust to living your life this way, and insurmountable challenges become doable.

However, if you feel like you need more help, I encourage you to seek help elsewhere and anywhere: friends, family, a gluten-free support group, or even a therapist or counselor. I know I did when I was diagnosed. There is absolutely nothing wrong with admitting that you need someone to talk to about this change and the struggles with adapting to a new diet and a new social life without gluten. *It might be exactly what you need.*

I thought after a few years that I totally nailed this thing. I saw some bloggers and authors who made it seem like their world had gone from black and white to color like in the *Wizard of Oz*. I want you guys to know that I'm still learning and still struggling, right along with you. Even when I see the Yellow Brick Road in front of me, sometimes these damn flying monkeys get in the way.

When I get glutened, I have to cope with more than just physical symptoms. When I start to feel any of the typical side effects, I try with all my might to recall where the hell I had gluten recently. Was it Chipotle? I thought I told them to change gloves and get new ingredients. Was it a new cookie I tried? Was something made on shared equipment that I didn't know about? Then my head spins from trying with all of my might to recall the last 10 days and everything that I've consumed. The anxiety is palpable. You know the drill; we've all gone through it a million times.

When I accidentally eat gluten, I tend to start feeling like dog crap. Inside my mouth, the usual giant ulcers develop. Although I wish I could maintain some sort of liquid diet while my flesh is ripped off the inside of my mouth like some sort of zombie, I can't resist eating real food. Anything salty is so painful that tears well up in my eyes. I am not able to eat well, or even talk well, and every time I open my mouth I'm in pain. Luckily I don't have many gastro symptoms, but man, does it bum me out. I've tried every remedy for aphthous ulcers, including several prescriptions. I tend to coat my sores with some miracle mouthwash (a combination of Benadryl, Maloxx, and Lidocaine). Like I told you earlier, I become a total sassy mess and am a pain to be with. I just sit in bed at night and roll my eyes in the dark and say, "Seriously celiac?!?!? Whyyyyyyy?"

I guess I'm writing this to tell you that even someone who is supposed to be an advocate—someone who is supposed to represent the needs and wants of a community, someone who completed all of the stages of grief—*still struggles* with what this disease does to my body. You are never alone out there; we all have our off days, and that's okay. You're allowed to cry. You're allowed to be mad. You're allowed to swear and rant about it on Facebook. You're allowed to scream out the car window, "IF I SEE ANOTHER GIRL SCOUT TROOP SELLING COOKIES I'M GONNA LOSE IT," as you travel from grocery store to grocery store trying to avoid their sales tactics.

Because, you know, that's probably how I feel too. Especially about the Girl Scouts.

That's one of the best things about the gluten-free community: we understand what we are going through. We all go through the emotional (and sometimes physical) withdrawal of gluten, and we understand the emotional perils of facing a lifelong gluten-free diet.

It does get better. It may take some time, but it will get better. Now get back to living your life free of those three jerks: wheat, rye and barley!

Why Celiac Is the Best Thing That Ever Happened to Me: Shooting Rainbows Out My Ass

---

In the introduction, I laid out five points as to why being diagnosed with celiac disease is the best thing that ever happened to me. Let's revisit and look in-depth at these five points (unless you skipped the introduction, in which case this is completely new information!).

1. I finally understand what's wrong with my body
2. My diagnosis gave me a game plan for the rest of my life
3. It's allowed me to meet so many new friends across the country whom I never would have met otherwise
4. It's a litmus test for friendship and relationships
5. It's given me a purpose in life: to educate and advocate

Number 1: I finally understand what's wrong with me

I'm not sure there's anything more annoying than having a medical problem that even a slew of doctors can't figure out. It's more annoying than being stuck in the express check-out lane with a person who has more than fifteen items. It's more annoying than being stuck in a traffic jam for hours with nothing good on the radio. It's more annoying than the feeling of stepping in cat barf early in the morning before you put on your glasses and you look down but you can't see anything but you know it's cat barf. I wondered for years what could be wrong with me—searching for a diagnosis, wanting to not feel crazy for feeling sick and weird and not normal for so long. It felt so good to have an answer.

Number 2: My diagnosis gave me a game plan

One of the best things about being diagnosed celiac or NCGS is that you have a game plan. For the rest of your life, you only have to do *one thing* to stay healthy. For the rest of your life, you only have to eat a gluten-free diet to get well. Okay, so that "only" is a big word with a lot of commitment and issues behind it, but consider the alternative. We (typically) don't have to take costly medications two or three times a day. We (typically) don't need injections, transfusions or transplants to stay well after diagnosis. Celiac is not a death sentence or a terminal illness.

While I think this is an awesome condition to have from that perspective, that's where the general community can get a little suspicious. "Wait, let me get this right You have a lifelong disease, but to 'cure' it you only have to eat gluten free?" It confuses the hell out of people. As a society, we're subjected to endless pharmaceutical ads on TV and in magazines, and we like to fix things with pills. I don't necessarily have a problem with that; medications have helped me through everything from gastroparesis to sinus infections. I'm not going to say that society is suspicious of a disease that is cured by food, but it definitely makes us "unique." At times, it even seems unbelievable to the general population.

I don't know about you, but I'd rather eat gluten-free than inject myself with an EpiPen and go to the ER or have regular transfusions. If I know the conditions I am pre-disposed toward, and I can manage my life around these risks. I know that if I eat gluten free, I can live a somewhat healthy and definitely happy life all on my own.

Number 3: Meeting new friends

"I'm a loner, Dottie, a rebel." The infamous line from *Pee Wee's Big Adventure* always kind of rang true with me. I've always had several good friends, but I'm not very good at making new friends. As much as I seem outgoing, I'm very private at times and love to stay at home alone and just watch movies. It doesn't help that Non-GFBF and I both love to cook at home, drink wine, and watch Netflix. We're both not anti-social, but I'd use the term "homebody" if it didn't have such a "we're cat people who don't like the outside world" connotation.

But being gluten free (especially becoming a gluten-free blogger) has turned my cat-lady life around and has forced me to meet new people. And guess what—I even liked it! At every expo I have met readers of my blog, which is amazing because sometimes I think it's just me (and my mom) reading my posts. I met amazing fellow gluten-free and food-allergy bloggers who are doing amazing things with their gift for writing. I bonded with people who I would have never met without this disease. I have forged unbreakable bonds and amazing relationships with people who live hours away from me across the country.

Number 4: A litmus test for relationships

Finding new friends (and yes, dating is a part of this) is hard for anyone, much less someone with a chronic illness, a food allergy, etc. Being "different" is often difficult, especially when you first meet someone and everyone is on his or her best behavior.

But being gluten free can also be a great litmus test for relationships and friendships. I would hate to think that someone could stop being my friend just because I have a different set of standards for how and what I eat. But as you can tell, some relationships can't handle the issues brought on by this disease.

After diagnosis, you'll be able to base relationships on a set of questions about understanding, empathy and compassion. Is this person a true friend or someone I want to spend my precious time with? Are they okay with understanding I might not want to go out if I'm feeling crappy? Will they understand that I always have to pick the restaurant, and if not, I might not eat there? Do they get when I have to call a venue ahead of time to see if they have anything safe for me to eat? What if we go back to the same restaurant over and over again because I know that they are safe? Will they eventually tire of me being special? Will they understand that I'm not just trying to get attention when I'm trying to order a safe meal?

These are all questions that I've heard during the many conversations I've had about celiac disease and being gluten free.

It's embarrassing, especially at first, to be the one with special needs. I see my friends going out to new restaurants all the time, and I wonder what that's like. What is it like to just go on Yelp and see what the hottest new place is and then go check it out? What would it be like to meet someone new and not talk about gluten? I don't even know what that's like anymore.

Luckily for me, I managed to find a decent guy who was willing to accept my gluten-free status, but also switch to a gluten-free diet, share a 100% gluten-free household with me, and help me run a gluten-free business. There will be more about my superstar in the chapter on dating. Needless to say, when I found him, I realized that my new lifestyle helped to sort the good from the bad.

And the same goes for friendships: the strong ones remained and thrived. My friends were always interested in what was new on my medical charts and genuinely engaged when I talked about celiac disease and any new research. They are fine when I pick the restaurant and understand that I may have anxiety over a new place. I don't think that I've lost any Facebook friends since posting all about my health issues—*I think*. You realize just how lucky you are to have people who support you through this journey, not tear you down or become annoyed that you are suddenly a "burden." You're not a burden; you're just different!

Number 5: Living with a purpose

Not that I was stumbling around aimlessly before I was diagnosed, but I really feel that I have a purpose now. I strive for celiac and NCGS education and advocacy every day. While some days I wish I could go an hour without using the word "celiac," it really is an honor to be imparting any of my gluten-free wisdom to those looking for it. My free time is spent reading countless articles about the disease, and attending educational events and conferences across the country. With so many damn myths about this subject, I feel like most of my day is spent on the Internet trying to keep the gluten-free hype machine from taking over the sanity of the natives.

I saw a Tumblr post a while ago, and it spurred my quest to look at the gluten-free lifestyle in as much of a positive a light as I could muster. I'm often bothered by the newly diagnosed (or those outside the GF community) who say stuff like, "I CAN'T HAVE ANYTHING ANYMORE EVER. I HATE YOU CELIAC! NO MORE BREAD OR PIZZA 4EVA!" This rant is typically followed by, "My life is terrible," "Now what," "F-this f-that, etc." I'm sure that these are the rants of someone who is grieving the loss of gluten.

Now, I totally understand the grieving process when it comes to gluten. I was taught to mourn the loss of gluten (like the prior chapter), and then move on and embrace my new healthy life. I could wallow in the pity and cry because it was the healthy thing to do, but then I had to get over it. However, when it comes to posts like this, I am the first to reassure them and say, "Yes, yes, you can have everything."

If I can help them move from grief and anger into acceptance—this is a success. If I can assure them that their life isn't over, it's a success. Now, that's not saying that the gluten-free counterpart to the product you're sad about tastes the same—it won't. Mourn the loss of that. I still mourn the loss of my favorite dish from Olive Garden (seriously, Olive Garden, why?), but I'm okay with that. I've learned to appreciate the direct substitutes that make my life easy while keeping me healthy (and alive).

Don't think I'm heartless or inhumane because of my anger when I see these posts. I remember being like that, so I do have empathy. I just feel like there's a lack of education about the quality of gluten-free substitutes that people don't understand. So, instead of having one ounce of happiness about a diagnosis, they just focus on what they can no longer eat, instead of seeing all the things they *can*.

I also get angry when I hear my friends say, "If I couldn't eat gluten, I would die." Why do people say that? We live in a society of such exaggeration: "OMG if I don't have that Marc Jacobs handbag, I will die!" Okay okay, I'm pretty sure I've said that before, *but* everything is some scientific permutation of "OMG . . . I'd die." Well, for many celiacs, we would die (or at least live a very, very sick life) if we continued to live in the world of wheat. I'm pretty sure if you shit your pants every time you ate a donut, friend, you wouldn't die if you had to eat gluten free. You'd probably be glad you don't have to squeeze your butt cheeks together tightly after every meal until you find the nearest bathroom. You'd shart your pants once, and I'm pretty sure you'd be okay with avoiding wheat again, friend—because if not, you might actually die of shame. Shart shame.

I used to be exactly like them. I used to tell people, "Oh yeah, that cookie is mine. You can tell it's gluten free because it's awful." And, "You don't want my gluten-free meal, it tastes terrible." Or when someone would say, "Is this gluten free?" and ask about an object that clearly had gluten in it, I joked, "Is it good? Then it has gluten in it. Gluten is what makes things tastes good." But I have challenged myself to stop perpetuating the myth that we eat sub-par foods. I assure you, we don't.

I often sit at the airport and see the rest of the world eating Cinnabons, Pizza Hut personal pan pizzas, french fries and burgers that are dripping everywhere, and I look at whatever stuff I packed and feel like I'm really eating healthier. I'm forced to pack, and I eat well: fresh fruit and veggies, KIND bars, GoPicnic snacks, popcorn, etc. I truly feel fortunate about the food I'm eating—sometimes to the point where I say to myself, "Man, I really would never go back to gluten even if I could." (Okay, sometimes I still really, really want a Cinnabon.)

I'm not sure if I'm the only one who feels this way, but that's honestly why I wanted to make an online gluten-free name for myself. I wanted to show people that there are products that taste good and are indeed gluten free! I laugh when coworkers ask, "Have you tried gluten-free pizza before?" and I say, "What kind?"—and I think they're a little shocked to see that there are options in our community. I like to kill the myth that we can't eat anything and instead perpetuate the stereotype that we have special food for us that can taste good too. I mean, sometimes it doesn't taste good—let's be honest—but I've had such good luck with products that I truly enjoy eating regularly and that are safe for me.

Even if your diagnosis of celiac or NCGS isn't the best thing that's ever happened to you, I hope that you can see the good in it. While there may not be rainbows shooting out of your ass yet, I hope you do grow to love the part of you that is healthier and that no longer has to guess why you were sick. And you can move forward on living a gluten-free life with a generally positive attitude (while being able to rant about Girl Scout cookies whenever you want—trust me, I'll support you).

First Timer Mistakes:
What I Learned and
What I Want to Teach You

If you're new to anything—a new language, a new job, a new relationship— you're bound to make mistakes. Making mistakes is just part of the learning process. However, there were so many mistakes to be made when I was first diagnosed that I'd like to share them with you now so you can easily avoid them. I want you to feel better as soon as you can!

Cross-contamination is real.

I don't know what the hell was wrong with me when I was first diagnosed. Maybe it's because I was simply told to "Google" the gluten-free diet and how to survive in this crazy world of wheat. Maybe it's because I didn't take celiac disease or gluten sensitivity seriously. Maybe I just was just stuck in the denial phase. Maybe I just wanted to be a badass. But regardless of the reason, for years I lived in a world where cross-contamination didn't exist. So, a crumb—A CRUMB—of gluten can cause a reaction in someone with celiac disease. AN ABSURDLY

TINY CRUMB! Like those tiny little things that fall out of a coworker's napkin after they disgustingly eat a bagel in front of you or those things at the bottom of the toaster in the kitchen. Those little things can really wreck you, and you should learn that from Day One of your diagnosis. I was taking croutons off of salads, prying apart the Starbucks breakfast sandwiches, and eating the McDonald's McSnack McWrap McRight out of the damn McWheatTortilla. I was an idiot. No wonder I wasn't feeling any better after going gluten-free! Although I wasn't eating bread, I was still getting glutened, like hardcore.

Wheat-free doesn't mean gluten-free.

Who the hell would make these products? Why? Okay, you're allergic to wheat—like a legitimate allergy—I understand. But isn't it just as easy to get a certified gluten-free product? Not only does it not have wheat, but it doesn't have all the other parts of gluten too. While I like to stick up for my only-wheat-free brethren, the rise of celiac disease and NCGS constitutes a huge market that could easily be confused by this labeling (I was when I was a n00b). Non-GFBF's mom was fooled into getting him a package of wheat-free cookies, because non-GF people associate "gluten" with "wheat." When they think about just "wheat," they stop paying attention to everything else, including hidden (or not so hidden gluten) such as barley malt. Speaking of wheat. . . .

Only wheat has to be labeled.

According to the Food and Drug Administration, *The Food Allergen Labeling and Consumer Protection Act* (FALCPA—or sometimes I refer to it as FALCOR because it's friendlier when I think of the dog from *The Never Ending Story*) is meant to "help Americans avoid the health risks posed by food allergens."

Wheat is one of the top (meaning most common, not the coolest) allergens, along with milk, eggs, fish, shellfish, tree nuts, peanuts and soybeans. However, this label only includes one part of the gluten trifecta, leaving out rye and barley. While I use the FALCPA statement to start, I read all of the ingredients and look for the tricky words that could potentially hide gluten in all its forms.

I will also look for the words "Gluten Free" on the label soon because this year, the FDA finally put their ruling into action on labeling "gluten free."[22] While this labeling law doesn't take effect until 2014, make it a habit to always read the ingredients. Every time. All the time.

"Gluten Free" and "Made Without Gluten Ingredients" don't always mean GF.

So currently companies can make claims that a product is gluten free without regulation. But maybe you're reading this after August 2014 and the FDA has settled all of this nonsense. Or maybe you're reading this on Google Glass ordering your jet pack off of eBay. I'm not saying that companies are out to get us and just want to put gluten in everything and say, "Ha, fooled you!" But, some people may not "get it" and claim that a product is safe to eat when it really isn't. And that puts us all in danger.

For example, I've had some negative experiences at farmers' markets. This fact bums the crap out of me. To me, farmers' markets are the most friendly and honest of all stores, right? You're meeting the people who are growing this food for you! It's so intimate! Which is why I hated

---

[22] As of August 5, 2014, labeling a product as "gluten free" must mean that product is under 20 ppm (parts per million) gluten. What is 20 ppm? Imagine looking at your piece of bread under a microscope and seeing all of the tiny parts that make up the bread. Out of a million particles, gluten would make up only twenty. Twenty ppm is the gluten-free standard, which means that all food labeled gluten-free *should* be less than that. But, it's not necessarily true for some products that just want to slap those words on their product for marketing. However, the jury is still out on this whole labeling law as the FDA is not *enforcing* testing. However, I really believe that we're headed in the right direction and eventually all food labeled gluten free will be safe for us. Yes, some minute percentage of the celiac population react to food under 20 ppm gluten, but these labeling laws are made for the majority of celiacs. And no, there is no such thing as testing for zero ppm of gluten—yet. If you want to live in a 0 ppm world, have fun in outerspace, eating in an astronaut suit. Have fun up there.

getting into a tussle with someone trying to sell non-GF oats as gluten free, and gluten-free food made in the same place as gluten food. It's just so frustrating. I'm lucky because my farmers' market has a farm that is full of celiacs—like seriously, the whole family is—and they make amazing gluten-free and GF vegan treats for the market. They also bring their baby goats, so that's a total plus if you sell me food that is safe to eat and I can pet a farm animal—win/win.

Just be careful with your health; I don't know how many times I have to say this to get through to people. If you're unsure about how a product is made, then don't eat it. If you do eat a food and have a reaction to it, stop eating it! Always read ingredients and always ask questions. Always be wary of products made in the same facility as wheat, and be very picky about products made on equipment shared with wheat (if you don't eliminate all of these products outright). Even though companies are supposed to have good manufacturing processes, if I don't trust my mom to clean surfaces in her home before I come over, I don't know why I trust a company to do it. I always look for a certification process (i.e., Gluten Intolerance Group's GFCO certification), which means a company has to care enough to earn that seal. A GFCO certification means that the product has been tested at 10 ppm or less. Some companies test their products to less than the standard (like 3 or 5 ppm), and proudly display this on their packaging and marketing. I always like to patronize the companies that go above and beyond when testing their products at a lower ppm.

Spelt, Emmer, Durum, Triticum, Einkorn, and Kamut are not Game of Throne characters; they are gluten and they are evil.

Well, they are all evil to us at least—if you are reading this book as a celiac or someone who can't eat gluten. There are so many versions and names for gluten—especially ancient wheat—that you always have to be on the lookout. However, I am happy that ancient grains are "so hot right now" because people are starting to bring these items to the forefront of food. This helps us because then people will start to understand what these things are. Parts of the ancient grain family that *are* safe are quinoa, sorghum teff, millet flax and amaranth. If you're not familiar with these safe grains, get to know them. They are awesome! One more thing that celiac gave to me: quinoa! Where would I be today without quinoa? I'd probably just be making regular rice in my rice maker instead of amazing coconut-milk-infused red quinoa. See, didn't that make me sound way cooler than just talking about rice?

Gluten is sneaky.

Gluten is sneaky and likes to hide everywhere. If you're not paying attention, there are many danger zones that may put a celiac at risk. I've listed some potential danger zones that you need to be wary of when living a gluten-free life.

Potential Household Danger Zone: The Bathroom

+ Gluten can hide in many body washes, soaps, lotions, creams and other beauty products. Although the gluten molecules are considered too big to pass through the skin according to the most recent celiac research, I know plenty of people who have gluten skin reactions. I also know that I get scalp sores much less using gluten-free hair products. Personally, I know how clumsy I am, and I'm sure that if I put something on my face, it will surely end up in my mouth somehow, so I avoid it topically too. My hair also does better with gluten-free shampoos and conditioners. And please, you know that you've had shampoo in your mouth, rushing around in the shower—I barely function at 6 a.m.

+ Lotion and hand sanitizers can contain gluten, and I recommend for everyone to give this up. Too often do I put lotion or sanitizer on my hand and then proceed directly to the kitchen for a snack. I don't want to develop more OCD tendencies than

I already have, so compulsive hand washing isn't an option for me. Opt for gluten-free lotion and sanitizer.

✦ Cosmetics are another source for gluten. Again, the experts say you only need gluten-free labeling on items that go in your mouth (like lipstick and lip balm), but I try to go gluten free just in case. If you wear facial make-up like a concealer or powder, I would encourage you to try a gluten-free brand and see if you notice any difference. I recommend Red Apple Lipstick for their gluten-free and paraben-free lipstick in killer shades like Rebel. Because no one said being a celiac couldn't be sexy.

Potential Household Danger Zone: The Kitchen

✦ The toaster is where all the Ghosts of Gluten Past live. Unless you want some sort of paranormal experience in your stomach, pitch your toaster and get a new one. However, you will soon realize that gluten-free toast is much smaller than regular toast. I was recommended to use toaster tongs to avoid burns. The scars on my hands are not from a badass street fight; they are from a hot toaster and Udi's bread.

✦ Everyone recommends getting a new colander when you are diagnosed because apparently no one in the universe has figured out how to properly clean a colander. Maybe in 2015.

✦ Wooden or porous anything is a no-no in the kitchen because it can absorb gluten. Start fresh with new kitchen items and knock yourself out at Bed, Bath, and Beyond.

Potential Household Danger Zone: The Medicine Cabinet

✦ Hopefully by the time you read this (or your children's children read this), there will be a law stating that drug manufacturers have to list any gluten in their medication. But (sigh), not yet. Until then, it's up to your detective skills and your patience with 1–800 numbers to find out if your medications contain gluten.

+ Utilize all resources available, including pharmacists and the online gluten-free community. Numerous sites compile online databases of gluten-free drugs, although I think the best one is glutenfreedrugs.com.

+ Nonprescription medication can also contain gluten, so make sure you're buying (and supporting) chains that label their gluten-free products, like Target and Walgreens branded items.

Potential Household Danger Zone: The Pets

+ Within the past year, we finally got the cats on a gluten-free diet. Many people don't think it's financially worth it to get their pets on a GF diet (as the food is often way more expensive and harder to find). However, for me it was all about peace of mind. The cats are constantly licking themselves, licking me, licking my food, drooling on my laptop. I don't want to have to dodge gluten from them too. I'd rather just put them on a grain-free diet and have them happily eating combinations of smelly tuna and whitefish and me feeling safe. Also, my snake was the OG pet in the house, as mice are naturally gluten-free.

Gluten Free can be a tax deduction.

If you are a diagnosed celiac, you can use your gluten-free food purchases as a tax deduction. However, there are many steps to the process, including tallying every single gluten-free item you've purchased during the year and comparing the price to the comparable non-GF item. Your deduction can include the difference between gluten-free food and gluten-full food. However, this deduction, along with your medical expenses, has to be a certain part of your income before you can use it as a deduction. See how confusing this can be? I already need a glass of (non-tax-deductible) wine just thinking about it. Consult the Celiac Disease Foundation's website and your tax preparer for more information on how to take full advantage of pricey gluten-free living.

I know that this information can be overwhelming at times, but try to approach this disease just one step at a time. Even though I'm years into my diagnosis, I still learn things every day about this disease and how to properly manage it. The key is to never stop learning and to glean knowledge from others who have been through the process so you don't have to repeat any of their mistakes.

Dining Out Part 1:
Learning to Trust the
Stranger Taking Your Order

"One cannot think well, love well, sleep well,
if one has not dined well."
—Virginia Woolf "A Room of One's Own"

Quit wincing; I promise the following chapters about dining out won't contain a single solitary sentence stating, "You can never dine out again." So many celiacs are terrified of dining out—and it's totally understandable. It's terrifying to put your own health into the hands of others. I totally get it. But, dining out is part of the American social tapestry. I couldn't give up gluten and give up dining out. Dining out is just far too important to me to get paranoid and stay home cooking for myself every day. Now, I'm not going to tell you that you can eat at every restaurant, and I'm not going to tell you to risk your health for the sake of being social. However, there are some places that are celiac friendly and safe for us.

Let's start with a dream scenario when dining out gluten free. Yes, I know there are a lot of "dream scenarios" in this book, but I think that understanding what is supposed to happen in the perfect world helps us navigate the imperfect world in which we live. If you *do* live in a perfect world where the following dream scenario happens every time you dine out, shoot me an e-mail and let me know if there are any condos for rent in your city. I'll be on the next flight out.

When you sit down to eat at a new restaurant, the server approaches you and says, "Welcome to Dream Kitchen USA. My name is Sergio. Can I take your order?" Since this is *my* dream, I'm also going to make the waiter super attractive, perhaps with a foreign accent and big puppy-dog eyes.

You say, gazing longingly into his eyes: "I have celiac disease. I don't know if you're familiar with it, but it's an autoimmune disease that causes terrible long-term harm to my body if I ingest even the smallest crumb of gluten—a protein found in wheat, rye, and barley."

Sergio chimes in, "Of course I know what celiac disease is. Here at Dream Kitchen USA, we are NFCA Great Kitchen program trained, and approved by the Celiac Sprue Association. Our staff is very well-informed about celiac disease and gluten-free dining, and we have regular training from our management down to our busboys on how to serve our gluten-free customers. We have a separate prep area, separate utensils and ingredients to assure no cross-contamination, and we serve our GF items on specially labeled plates so that you can tell when your food has been especially prepared just for you."

He adds, "Also, I'm single, but I know you have a boyfriend, so I'm offering to come clean your house shirtless for free, because I understand that you've been going through a difficult time since your diagnosis."

If you've ever tried to dine gluten free you know that you'd be slapping yourself awake right now if this experience happened to you. Even as a blogger, no one has offered to clean my house once.

Next, you order off the gluten-free menu (which is separate from the other menu *of course*), which clearly states that each item is gluten free, and labels other potential allergens as well. The menu describes to you what exactly is in each item and/or where it is from.[23] The menu has great substitutes, like a burger with a gluten-free bun instead of just offering their burger on a lettuce cup. They also indicate that they have a separate fryer for their fries that is regularly cleaned! You order the burger and fries combo and send Sergio back to the kitchen to relay your order, with the word "allergy" scribbled all over it so the back of the house knows that it's a serious condition.

Sergio's runner delivers the specialty plates to your table and repeats the order exactly as you ordered it, adding that it is gluten free. Every time someone drops off a plate, regardless of what it is, they alert you that it is gluten free.

Sergio's manager comes out to greet you mid-meal and asks how everything is. He says he likes to check in on his "special" customers and make sure that your dining experience meets your needs. He is excited about catering to the gluten-free population because it directly affects his bottom line! He knows that one in 133 people have celiac disease and even more have gluten intolerance, and he knows he has to treat those people right because he also knows that word of mouth is quick in our community. You leave the meal satisfied, having eaten some of the best GF buns you've ever had. *And then you wake up.*

Since going gluten-free, I've had a few "perfect" scenarios, although most of them were at dedicated gluten-free restaurants and bakeries. Rarely does this scenario happen outside of those places, but I know in my heart that it exists. On the plus side, many of the restaurants I've been to have *some* iteration of this dream sequence. I've been fortunate to visit a lot of restaurants that do gluten free right. I've also had experiences that have scared the crap out of me, and subsequently—in a week

---

[23] For example, I would love if a restaurant told me that their gluten-free buns are made down the street at a gluten-free dedicated bake shop and would then list the potential allergens in them (dairy, eggs, soy), so I would feel more confident in my choices. I'd also love for their gluten-free buns to not taste like shit, if at all possible.

or so— I woke up with mouth sores, and I cursed the sky because I have no idea which of the shady experiences truly did me in.

Let me run down some do's and don'ts of dining gluten-free[24].

CHOOSING A RESTAURANT:
DO: Use Yelp and other review sites

Visit Yelp.com, Urbanspoon and other local online review sites to find restaurants that claim to be gluten free. Then do some digging into what they offer and how friendly they are for specific diets. I also like to get a good vibe of a restaurant's customer service from sites like these. If a restaurant is rude to a "normal" diner, imagine how they will be with someone with a specialty diet!

Sometimes I get really lucky and I find a review from a fellow celiac or gluten-intolerant diner—but that's pretty rare. I have to scour a ton of reviews in order to find one like that. But, I always encourage people with specialty diets to leave reviews on these sites and pay it forward for the next special diner.

Yelp is a great place to connect with other gluten-free people too—especially people in your same city. You'll get to see where they eat safely and read their reviews if you "friend" them on the social network. If you have the app, you can also leave "tips" for friends, and I like to leave snippets about a restaurant's gluten-free menu.

DO: Search blogs for reviews

Sometimes there's nothing quite as easy as using smart search terms with a search engine like Google. "Gluten Free Phoenix" for instance, yields some results that I didn't even know (and I live there) from bloggers.

---

[24] When I say "gluten-free dining," I mean dining with the mindset that gluten is rat poison. If you're just eating gluten-free for shits and giggles, you don't have to pay such close attention to anything I say here, but then again, I'm not really sure why you're reading this book if gluten doesn't make you as sick as my cat was after consuming half a basil plant we intended for pasta night. Yes, that actually happened. And he threw up a whole basil leaf. Impressive.

Although I'd love to say that you should be loyal to certain bloggers (because we love to have loyal fans), using search terms will help you find more places in which you can dine safely. I've found several new blogs via search terms, and I know that many people have found my own blog through searching. Personally, some of my favorite blog posts I've posted have been posts about our travels, where I've reviewed restaurants during our vacations. How did I find some of those restaurants? Other bloggers! See how that works?

Keep in mind that the older the blog post, the more likely the restaurant has updated its menu—which might mean a change in their gluten-free offerings. Always check with a restaurant for their gluten-free offerings, even after reading a recent restaurant review.

DO: Use gluten-free dining apps and websites

There are many apps and websites outside of Yelp that allow gluten-free consumers easy access to gluten-free-friendly restaurants and consumer-generated reviews. It seems like I see new apps pop up frequently, but I'm a heavy user of two sites that I consider invaluable to gluten-free diners:

- CanIEatHere.com website
  - Helps you identify restaurants in your area that are suitable for people with food allergies and/or are eating gluten free, vegan, or kosher.
  - Based on communal reviews
  - Supported by paid advertisements and sponsorships (featured listings)
- FindMeGlutenFree.com website and app
  - Helps you identify gluten-free restaurants in your area
  - Easily accessible via phone app
  - Only searches for gluten
  - Based on communal reviews
  - Supported by paid advertisements and sponsorships (featured listings)

There are multiple apps that focus on fast-food menus and that try to keep them as up to date as possible. Other apps focus on foods within restaurants and help you decide the safest food to eat in any restaurant.

DO: Read the menu before you go in

Non-GFBF always thinks it's a buzz kill to know what he is going to order before he goes into a restaurant. I, however, don't have another option. It's our duty to take our safety into our own hands (until our smart order reaches the kitchen, and then we hope and pray the chef knows what the hell he or she is doing).

What I learned in Girl Scouts (besides how many Thin Mints I could shove in my mouth at one time) was to always be prepared. Or maybe I learned that from some cute Boy Scouts? Regardless, it's your duty to be prepared before you get into a restaurant. There are a few things I look for on a restaurant's website:

1. A gluten-free menu OR gluten free marked on the menu (either gluten free or RGF—request gluten free). This is a sign they know what they're doing.
2. Some sort of food allergy/intolerances/specialty diet section or paragraph. I want a restaurant that prides itself on knowing what they're doing—so much so that they want to publicize it and talk about it. Maybe it's a story about how they understand the needs of special guests like gluten free or food allergies. Maybe it's a story about their special prep area for their gluten-free pizza (again, a *dream* scenario).
3. A menu with all of the ingredients listed for each menu item. God bless America when there is a menu item that includes all of its ingredients so I don't have to guess. What's in your sandwich? Do you have croutons on your salad? What the hell is in that sauce?

When I call a restaurant, I address all the things that I just mentioned. However, you have to be prepared that the person who answers the phone may not know what they're talking about. The person who kindly answered the phone may just be taking reservations, and might not even spell your name accurately. If you ask them about a gluten-free menu and they sound panicked (you can easily tell if it's panic, even if there is silence on the other end of the phone), ask for a manager. Now, if the manager doesn't know, you should probably choose another restaurant.

ORDERING
DO: First announce your allergies

Sometimes I forget that I'm different (and not in that "isn't she special—we should give her a trophy for something we made up to make her feel like a champion" way). Some days, for a few hours, I can *actually* forget that I eat differently than other people. When I sit down at a restaurant, especially one that I've dined at a million times before, I forget that I am a special diner. When I order the pizza, of course I order the gluten-free pizza—obviously. *Wait, did I order the gluten-free pizza?* Yeah, sometimes I guess I want to be "normal" so much that I actually forget to announce my dietary restrictions. When the waitress brings an obviously gluten-full pizza to the table, I sheepishly look up at her with the biggest puppy-dog eyes I can muster and say, "Uhhhh, I actually need that to be a gluten-free pizza." Of course, I offer to pay for it (and luckily they haven't taken me up on that offer yet) and apologize profusely. It's not their job to know my food allergies, even if I have it tattooed on my forehead (which I don't recommend for anyone who wants a professional career in the future). Don't be me! Always announce how special you really are!

After the server introduces himself/herself and gives the daily download of specials, this is your time to speak up. Since you've already studied the menu, or are holding a gluten-free menu in your hand, you're prepared.

Tell the server that you have celiac disease. I follow that up with an announcement that it is an allergy to gluten. *Yes, I say "allergy."* I know it's not scientifically accurate. I know that people with celiac disease don't like it when people call their autoimmune condition an allergy. However, in the food-service industry, everyone is trained on (or *should* be trained on) food allergies—no one wants to have an anaphylaxis incident in their restaurant. Most understand that a peanut allergy is life-threatening, and although it wouldn't hurt me immediately if I was accidently served a crouton, I know that it would render long-term damage if I was served carelessly on a frequent basis. But, I also know that our sensitivities all vary. I met a woman who has seizures—yes *grand mal* seizures—when she is given gluten. Can you imagine if you were the owner of a restaurant and a patron had a seizure in your dining room? Unforgiveable. So sometimes I bend science a little to get my point across. I tell them that I will get very, very, very (extra very's) sick if I am given anything with gluten in it.

DO: Talk to the manager

Now, maybe you're lucky and just after you went into the above speech, you found out that the server was very knowledgeable about the gluten-free lifestyle and about the seriousness of celiac disease. However, if your server seems even the slightest bit clueless or flippant about your requests, you need to ask to talk to the manager.

Go through the whole procedure again with the manager. By God, at this point if no one knows what you are talking about, I'll give you the same advice—RUN! Hopefully the manager knows what he or she is doing and will match you up with a server who better understands your needs or will address your special order himself/herself. At least, a good manager who cares about good reviews and repeat guests will do that.

DO: Ask about cross-contamination procedures

Outside of celiac and NCGS, there is a huge increase in the popularity of the gluten-free diet. It has become a gluten-free fad. Gluten-free "diet" is consistently ranked as a top marketing trend and "hot menu" trend for the restaurant industry. There are some (not all) restaurants that just want to keep up with the trends and demands of fickle diners.

So, they adopt a gluten-free menu, but may not do so wholeheartedly. Perhaps they understand that they can't offer gluten buns or pasta only, and maybe they've even ordered a direct substitute for the product like wholesale GF buns or rice pasta. *But unfortunately, for most it stops there.*

Restaurants may not quite understand exactly how sensitive a celiac is to contamination. They figure, "Hey, if we can just give someone an item prepared on our line that doesn't have big chunks of bread in it, we're good—right?" *No, not right at all.*

Have you seen a kitchen—like actually been inside of one? Have you seen a prep area? It's terrifying for a celiac. I don't want to scare you into not dining out, but I do want to scare you enough to ask about proper procedures when it comes to cooking something *on* the gluten-free menu.

Things where shit gets real in the back of the house:

+ Eggs and pancake batter. Seriously? SERIOUSLY. Who the hell decides that God-made packets of chicken babies aren't good enough? Well, the people at IHOP did. As of a few years ago (and currently) they add pancake batter to their omelets to make them fluffier. Who wants an egg pancake? Not me—that's *not* what I ordered. Granted, I would not walk into an IHOP and assume that they have a gluten-free menu, but the point of the story is that you never know what kind of screwed-up versions of real food people can put on a menu. When you order eggs, ask what's in it. I know it sounds ridiculous, and you'll sound ridiculous at every place that *doesn't* put pancake batter in their eggs, but it's better that you check. Also, eggs are often cooked in butter on a griddle. I ask for my eggs to be cooked separately in a fresh pan so there's no weird griddle contamination—same for any bacon I may order. Now, if the universe starts putting pancakes on my bacon without my knowledge, I'm going to be pissed.

+ Gluten-free toast can mistakenly be prepared in a gluten-full toaster. My practice is to not order gluten-free toast at a restaurant unless they offer it via toast bags or they assure me that they have a gluten-free labeled toaster that is special for celiac guests (fat chance getting that). I suppose they can make toast in a separate pan, but unless you're getting grilled cheese between your toast, just get a side of fruit, and you'll probably be happier.

+ Gluten-free pancakes can mistakenly be made on the same griddle as regular pancakes. Ask for your pancakes to be prepared on a separate pan that has been thoroughly cleaned.

+ Gluten-free pasta can mistakenly be boiled in the same water that just contained gluten-based pasta. Ask for your pasta to be prepared in a fresh pot of water, and ask for a gluten-free colander to be used to strain the pasta.

+ Gluten-free pizza is a difficult one, so I recommend you get your pizza from a restaurant that has been trained thoroughly, or you might end up with a Domino's problem (safe crust, unsafe environment). You'll have to ask for your pizza to be prepared separately—away from the other pizza and certainly not on the same prep line as gluten pizza. If they make the dough from scratch, the dough has to be prepared separately from the other pizza dough and away from any airborne flour used in the process of making the gluten pizza. Ask for separate (and new) sauce and ingredients from the back using separate ladles. The pizza needs to be cooked on a pizza stone that does not touch the same surface as a gluten pizza. I know: it sucks *all* of the fun out of pizza!

+ Anything grilled on the same surface as gluten can make you sick! It's crazy the things that I've seen grilled next to each other (and on top of each other). The grill is like a crazy orgy of gluten: you never know what remnants of past gluten parties you'll pick up when you have your safe food grilled on there. Hopefully the restaurant you're at keeps a separate part of the grill separate for gluten-free items. If not, ask for your stuff to be grilled on a separate pan.

DO: Ask to alter the menu for safety

No one will judge you if you ask to omit things that might be sketchy. Go ahead, girl—order whatever you want. I used to be afraid of changing the menu to fit my dietary needs, and now I say *screw it*. If they don't want to take my money and my When Harry Met Sally-like intricate orders, then clearly I don't need to be spending my hard-earned money at that joint.

WHEN THE FOOD ARRIVES
DO: Ask if every dish put on the table is gluten free

This seriously grinds my gears. If I order a gluten-free item, I need you to reassure me that the item you bring me twenty minutes later is, indeed, gluten free. I know that a lot can happen in twenty minutes. I want to make sure that whatever the hell you've been doing for twenty minutes didn't include confusing my order with one that has gluten in it. This is particularly annoying when a runner is involved. I feel like the intimate bond that I just made with the server when I spent ten minutes detailing what to do with my customized order has been broken. I feel let down, like at the end of a date when the guy doesn't ask when he can see you again. I feel like standing up and running to the kitchen and shouting at the server, pulling on her apron string and saying, "DOES WHAT WE HAD MEAN NOTHING TO YOU?" But I don't.

When the runner sets the food down, ask them if it is gluten free. Again, if they seem hesitant to answer, or look at you with eyes that dart back and forth like they are giving you a tell during an important hand of poker, ask to have the server come back. Just have someone assure you that whatever he or she brought out is what you needed and is safe to eat. If all else fails, have someone ask the chef who actually made your food. It's happened before to me; I've had to go all the way up the food chain to the person who actually prepared my food. It wasn't easy, and it took an annoying amount of time, but it was worth it.

DO: Inspect the food

So you have this beautiful plate of food in front of you. It's time to dive in, right? Wrong. Time to play Sherlock Holmes with your dish (I originally wrote "Angela Lansbury" but feared no one would know who that was). Does it look like the item you ordered? Awesome, that's the first step. I like to do a visual inspection to see if what's on the plate matches the description of the item. Is there any foreign sauce that wasn't listed? If so, that could be a hidden source of gluten.[25] Are there any unexpected garnishes on it?[26] It's these last-minute details—which seem to get left out of menus or forgotten about in the back of the house—that you need to pay attention to.

DO: Keep food safe from any gluten

So your meal has now passed the test—time to protect it. I'm not telling you to hoard your food like you're one of those doomsday preppers, or to guard your food like you just got out of prison. I'm just telling you to keep an eye on it. If your dining friends are not eating gluten free, there's a chance your food can get contaminated.

I was never one of those girlfriends who *shared* meals with my ladies on Friday nights—where everyone orders ten appetizers and eats off of everyone else's plates and gab about life. *I'm not into that.* I have always received terrible looks when I tell people that I don't share at restaurants—even before going gluten free, before I had a good reason to do so. I want *my* meal. I don't want *your* meal or else I would have ordered it.

Now I have a good reason to not want to share meals. First off, whomever I'm with (besides my guy) is probably not gluten free so

---

[25] This happens to me at new sushi joints when I forget (yes, it happens to everyone) to ask about the sauce. When the awesome roll comes out with a ponzu sauce, I am heartbroken and have to send it back. My sushi joint likes to sneak soy sauce into all of their sauces, so if it's liquid and it comes out on my fish, I always have to question it.

[26] It seems to happen to me at fancy restaurants that they just have to put some sort of crostini in my perfectly fine gluten-free food, and then I get all huffy about it. And at my gelato place: what are these people doing shoving a cookie into my perfectly fine cup of egg-yogurt?

there's gluten all over their business. Then, to get items off of my safe plate, they're using their utensils that have touched gluten. No thank you. This is especially important if you have any shareable items—like dips and sauces—as these items can be dipped into or dispensed with a communal utensil. Sharing guacamole is fine, as long as all of the chips are gluten free and there is no double-dipping (c'mon, be a gentleman). Sharing a spread is harder to do, but nothing is impossible. Just try to serve yourself first, and don't go in for seconds later.

This also goes for sharing drinks, which I'm super grossed out about anyways. Backwash and lip-to-lip contact is a no-no unless you're both eating and drinking gluten free, and the other party didn't sneak in a piece of bread while you weren't watching.

WHEN YOU GET THE CHECK:
DO: Tip well

As you know, servers depend on their tips to survive. I know there are some crappy ones in the bunch, but it's like that with any profession! When you get a good server, you've got to thank them for it. You can thank them by giving them at least a 20 percent tip.

DO: Give Feedback

Was there a way for this restaurant or this server to serve gluten-free patrons better? Was there something that could be improved, or something you'd like to see in the future? After you've thanked the server, ask to talk to the manager and tell them that you have some feedback on how to work with gluten-free diners.[27] I honestly believe that restaurants *want* to learn and want to try to do better and want to serve their patrons. At least, from my reasoning the equation is more

---

[27] If you don't feel like being ballsy during dinner—especially if you have delayed sensitivity and you don't know if you actually got sick yet. You can follow up with them via e-mail or social media (privately—don't slam them on their Facebook page unless they were real a-holes).

happy customers = more loyal customers = more money! If I owned a restaurant, that's what my goal would be!

By providing feedback, you're paying it forward for future diners. This is a great way to help out the gluten-free community while also raising (correct) gluten-free awareness at restaurants.

Dining Out Part 2:
What If I Work in a Restaurant?

Now, I know that the majority of the people who purchased this book won't be the ones who really need to read it. That would just be *too perfect*. But, I feel like I would be missing out if I didn't put a section in here for those of you who: a) own a restaurant; b) work in a restaurant; c) have connections to the restaurant or food and beverage industry. You guys are the ones who handle our food and therefore you are very important to me. You are in charge of my food, and you are the one standing in the way of me getting ill. Don't you feel powerful now? *You should.*

While people in the food-service industry are required to get permits and are trained in food safety, that's where the education usually stops. And while many are trained on food allergies, I believe much more education is needed for specialty diets and what a true gluten-free meal requires.

I'm fortunate enough to dine at some high-end restaurants. While I often make food at home, Non-GFBF and I live in a culinary hotbed. We have so many restaurants near us that are local focused and boutique. Fortunately for us, most of them understand gluten-free dining and do everything they can to keep me safe when I go in for a meal. I usually drop between $40 and $60 for a meal for two. Because I'm paying that amount of money, I assume that my food will be prepared expertly, safely, and the way I want it. But, you probably know that assumptions make an "ass" out of "u" and me.

In my short life as a celiac, I've been served gluten-full instead of gluten-free food several times. Now, only once have I been served regular pasta instead of GF pasta. However, other times I've been served items that I was assured were GF, but were not—like items fried in the same fryer as gluten, items cooked on the same surface as gluten, etc. While I want to shake these servers and managers and slap them across the face for getting me sick, perhaps I should blame the lack of education instead of resorting to fantasized violence. Maybe they just don't know. *And that's the scary part.*

Restaurants are using gluten free as a huge marketing trend—which leads to more choices for us, but also should *worry us.* Too often do I see celiacs get so excited about the gluten-free fad diet trend because they say it gives them more options. That's awesome—only if the restaurants know how to do gluten free properly. Too many of them (even the ones that think they are going to be trendsetters by adopting a GF menu) get us very sick because they don't know how to do it *right.*

Here are some of my tips for the food industry.

FIRST, UNDERSTAND WHAT GLUTEN REALLY IS:

These are things I've heard at restaurants I've dined at. I know, I can't stop shaking my head either.

"You can't have it, it has rice in it."—Why does everyone assume that rice is gluten? I don't even understand how that *myth* got started.

"That roll isn't gluten free because it's topped with sriracha."—If Sriracha had gluten in it, I'd be *very, very sad.*

"This has gluten in it, because it's made with whey."—Sweet Jesus, whey is milk, *not wheat.*

"The chips and guacamole are gluten free because the chips are corn."—Which sucks, because most likely those chips are cooked in the same fryer as gluten, so, sigh—*they are wrong.*

"That sauce just has a little bit of flour in it, is that okay?" No.

"Our ponzu sauce just has a little soy sauce." Well then it's a little bit *not at all* gluten free.

Gluten is a protein. It is found in wheat, rye, and barley and all of the fun derivatives of those. Gluten is in many things besides just pasta, bread and croutons. Gluten is also commonly used as filler and can be found in ingredients like your sauces, dressings and seasonings. It can also be found in candy, natural flavoring, and anything else that you have in your kitchen that is delicious. But *seriously*, if you're going to take gluten-free dining seriously, you first need to identify where gluten hides in your kitchen. Once you know, everyone on your staff should know too. If one person isn't aware or doesn't know enough to avoid making someone sick, your whole restaurant is affected.

FRONT OF HOUSE IS THE FIRST LINE OF DEFENSE:

I went to a blogger dinner once, and the waiter assured us that the chips were gluten-free. It wasn't too far-fetched; after all, the chips were made from corn.[28] But what really got me is when we asked about the way they were prepared—and where they were fried. We were assured that they were gluten free and prepared in a separate fryer. Victory was ours.

After we had eaten some of these chips, we were transferred to another table with another server. When this server ran down what we could and could not have on the menu (because she actually knew what she was talking about—a novel concept), we inquired about ordering more chips and guacamole. The server then informed us that we couldn't order the chips because they had gluten. Yep, those gluten-free

---

[28] If you ignore the fact that corn is all Frankenstein and GMO-ey (a subject I could rant on, but I'll save that for a later date), corn is "kosher" for us. Please don't subscribe to corn cross-reactivity myths! However, you can be "sensitive" to corn.

chips weren't so gluten-free because the gluten-free fryer was definitely not gluten free.

My eyes grew wide, and my jaw dropped. UGH. The rumbling started in my stomach—not because I ate the chips, but because members of our group did, and I was so alarmed that someone had lied to us! I was so sick to my stomach that I wouldn't have continued with the meal, should it not have been fully paid for by the PR firm we were there with. Not that a sponsored dinner makes it okay—and it wasn't—but we stayed on the roller-coaster ride so we could report back what could be fixed in the restaurant to make it ready to serve the next gluten-free guest. We paid it forward and paid in stomach upset.

Front of house—the staff who face the customer, are the only ones we *typically* get to talk to. Let's start with the guy who didn't know what he was talking about. Dear Mr. "Let's Guess and Be an A-Hole": By assuring us that the fryer is separate, you made several people ill. If you do not know if they are fried separately, ASK FIRST. Do not assume. Check daily with the chef and kitchen staff to make sure that everything is up to date and that the front-of-house knows what "daily specials" contain allergens.

UNDERSTAND CROSS-CONTAMINATION AND WHAT IT DOES TO US:

For those who have a hard time understanding the concept of cross-contamination, I like to use the rat-poison metaphor. If you let a few sprinkles of rat poison into an entrée, you'd get people pretty sick. And what a terrible PR move for the restaurant, right? Could you imagine all the Yelp reviews after that? You'd need a *Kitchen Nightmares* Gordon Ramsey-esque intervention to recover from that one.

You have to think of gluten as rat poison to our unique bodies. When we tell you that we have a serious reaction to gluten, you need to identify where you keep the rat poison and how to keep it away from our dishes.

Cross-contamination can occur via these three circumstances:

+ **Hands to ingredients.** If any of your back-of-house is using hands or gloves to touch an ingredient containing gluten, their hands are contaminated. There can be gluten crumbs all up in there and hands should be washed and/or gloves should be changed before preparing a gluten-free meal. When your hand or glove touches a gluten-containing ingredient and then later touches a safe ingredient—congratulations, you've contaminated that ingredient too. Think about Chipotle and the prep line scenario. If your Chipotle burrito maker is touching the flour tortilla and then grabbing lettuce and cheese by the handful and throwing it on the flour tortilla all willy-nilly (there's that word again), what about all those crumbs of flour that are all over the lettuce and cheese? Yes, it's that intense, folks. Ask for fresh gloves to be used and fresh ingredients too.

+ **Utensils to ingredients.** Think about a sauce ladle on pizza. You will probably touch the ladle to the pizza dough when spreading the sauce, right? That's the only way to really get it spread around in a circle, right? Well, that ladle and sauce touched gluten (assuming you're not at an all-GF pizza place). Once you put the ladle back into the sauce, it's contaminated. And what about a spoon used to stir gravy that's also used to stir a gluten-free sauce? Thanks for all the flour, dudes! Ask for different utensils and different ingredients to be used!

+ **Surfaces to ingredients.** Like we talked about before, wood surfaces such as cutting boards are a no-no, along with other porous surfaces. If you're preparing gluten-free meals in your kitchen, have a separate prep station that never gets used to prepare gluten-containing food. If you're cooking in a pizza oven, don't prepare the gluten-free pizza on the same surface you cook gluten pizza! Get a dedicated pizza stone! Grills at restaurants kill me (metaphorically of course, although only a slight exaggeration in reality, as they can make me very sick). Let me tell you a little story of an upscale boutique eatery by our house. In fact, as I type this sentence, I'm enjoying an Americano there right now. They introduced a gluten-free pizza a little while back and I went apeshit over it. Non-GFBF and I were dining there two or three times a week, and I couldn't get enough of it. We loved it so much that we even convinced our friends to stop eating the gluten crust and switch to the gluten-free crust. But, then I started getting continuously sick. We figured that it was the pizza and stopped eating for a while. I was incident-free for a few months, and then we decided to try the restaurant again and just skip the pizza. We had a few appetizers like the grilled caprese plate and the grilled artichoke with their quinoa salads. One day we sat at the chef's table, which positioned me with a direct line of sight into the open kitchen. As I was staring off aimlessly into the distance, I realized that I was looking at the grill, and then I realized what exactly I was looking *at*. I was looking at my tomatoes and my artichoke halves, face down on a grill. Then I saw all of the other items right next to my meal on the grill, like bread and the wings covered in gluten-full barbecue sauce. *Oh, now I get it.* It was the items on the menu I wasn't worried about that got me sick, not the giant blatantly-obvious gluten pizza of death. We pulled the server aside and told him that he needed to let the staff know about the grill situation. We've been back, but I haven't ordered a pizza or anything grilled in a long time. As a restaurant, you should have a dedicated section of the grill for gluten-free items, or cook them in separate pans or skillets.

DO NOT TRIVIALIZE THE AMOUNT OF CROSS-CONTAMINATION YOU DO HAVE:

Let's think back to the gluten-free-no-wait-they-are-contaminated-just-kidding chip situation we talked about earlier in this chapter. Once the manager found out that we had been glutened by their chips, they made the comment, "Hope you didn't eat a lot." Seriously? Why wouldn't you want us to eat and enjoy the food that you should be proud to serve? It also doesn't matter if you had one chip or the entire bowl—gluten is gluten, buddy. Again, it doesn't matter if you put one gluten item in a fryer, it's contaminated now, and you can't tell us that you're using a separate fryer. Please don't lie to appease us; we'll get sick and know about it! Gluten sees through your lies, and into your deep fryer, friends.

ALERT PATRONS OF INGREDIENTS:

I know this one is a wish-list item, but damn—there are so many food intolerances and specialty diets nowadays that I think smart restaurants should label their menus. I'm not just talking about gluten free. Restaurants need to label vegetarian and vegan items. By putting an alert on your menu for these diets, you're announcing that you are friendly to that particular group. And who doesn't need a friend?

My dream is to live in a world where all menu ingredients are included on a menu. Or at least give us a general idea of what's in there. Like guacamole—label it if there's cheese on it. If there's a salad, tell us if it comes with croutons so we know to order without it.

WHEN YOU KNOW YOU DID SOMETHING WRONG, ADMIT IT, AND THEN MAKE IT UP TO ME:

Continuing on with our earlier fiasco with the chips, if I were the one who ate the chips I would have thrown a fit. I'm not good about that stuff in public. As Non-GFBF will tell you, I have lost my shit numerous times in public because of something really dumb that a restaurant has done in regards to gluten. Although the chip server did apologize, he never really asked *how* we were feeling, or what he could do to make it better. Oh man, if I was the manager and I screwed up that badly and made someone ill, I would do the following things to attempt to make it right:

1. Seriously apologize. Not the type of apology where you say, "I'm sorry you feel that way." No one likes those types of apologies,

and everyone sees through them. Genuinely feel bad about what you and your restaurant staff have done in error.

2. Bring the chef out to see me to apologize for the miscommunication. Have him or her talk about the procedures typically in place to avoid incidents like this in the kitchen. Even though it may not be the chef's fault, at least it saves the restaurant's face.

3. Then, I'd offer the person who got ill—and everyone affected by it (the rest of the dining party that has to deal with the emotional shenanigans you now put their friend through)—a hefty gift card to encourage them to dine with you again, where you try to make it up next time. Be prepared for the patron to decline the offer; after all, you made them sick the first time so what would make them think you're going to do better the next time. I've turned down a "sorry we screwed up" gift card only one time, and that's because I didn't trust the restaurant to not screw up a second time. Trust is hard to rebuild with the community once it has been broken, so a) try not to screw up in the first place, and b) attempt to rectify the situation as kindly and quickly as possible.

4. You should also offer to give the diner a tour of the kitchen and walk us through proper kitchen protocols that you typically implement or will be implementing to avoid this situation again. Or ask to sit down with us and understand OUR needs and how other patrons like us won't get sick at your place.

MAKE GLUTEN-FREE DINING EASY FOR US AND THE FRONT OF HOUSE:

At the gluten chip place, they didn't mark GF or GF-friendly menu items on the menu. Instead, the servers had to rely on memory as to which part of the dish had gluten in it (and therefore had to be subbed out) or what dishes were naturally gluten free. Of course, it's terrifying when everything coming out of a server's mouth is, "Uhhh, I think that's gluten free, but let me check." I love that you're checking every five minutes with the chef, honey, but please know ahead of time what things are safe without giving us the blank expressions of a doe about to be tackled by a Chevy truck.

Mark your menu items with a GF or RGF—request gluten free. Make notes about what needs to be subbed on each dish to make it friendly. Put these notes on the menu or on a piece of paper that servers can carry around. That way patrons can feel safe about ordering a dish, and servers don't have to look like they don't know what they're doing. Make it easy for them to make us feel at home while dining.

PAY ATTENTION TO HOW THE DISH IS ORDERED:

With the chip experience, there were only six of us—in my opinion, a manageable party for any experienced server. One of our patrons, however, wasn't gluten free. That should be easy, right? Everyone is a weirdo except one. This guy ordered a dish that *could* be made gluten free by subbing out one ingredient. He asked for the gluten-containing ingredient on the side so he could enjoy the dish in its entirety and the other diners could enjoy the safe, gluten-free version of the dish. On top of all of their other missteps—the entrée came out in one piece, with no side dish, and was placed on the table without warning that it was a gluten-containing dish.

If we ask for something on the side, we mean it. If the entire table is gluten free, except for one person—take note of that. Make sure the food runners know that this dish is special and needs to be announced as such. The entire table was sharing off of each other's dishes. Should I not have known that the dish was gluten, I would have gone Incredible Hulk on someone.

MY PERSONAL NEW PET PEEVE IS FLOURLESS CHOCOLATE CAKE WITH FLOUR:

Seriously. After an already crappy meal with the chip shenanigans, we received the dessert menu. The server told us the only thing on it we could have was sorbet. Please note that the *other* item on the menu was a *flourless* chocolate cake. We all scratched our heads thinking—um, flourless? Why would a flourless cake contain gluten? But just like you've read throughout the book so far, you can't make assumption. The server checked with the chef and came back to tell us, "The cake has gluten throughout." Wait, a flourless chocolate cake with gluten? Way to confuse gluten-free guests! I just put my hands to my head and sighed.

As my final note to restaurants, if you are going to say you're friendly to gluten-free diners, please do it right.

If you don't want to serve us, you don't have to, but if you want our discretionary income (and there's a lot of us out there), please do it right. And don't be the a-hole that has flourless chocolate cake with flour in it.

Dining Out Part 3: Examples of Situations Where I Wanted to Punch Someone in the Face

If you're already afraid of dining out, perhaps you should skip this chapter. Asking you to read this chapter would be like asking your kid to watch *Paranormal Activity* with you and then sending him off to bed alone. These stories are *not* here to serve as scare tactics to discourage you from dining out, only things that I've learned after many *many* (sometimes hilarious) mistakes.

I'LL HAVE THE OVERPRICED SIDE OF GLUTEN *SI VOUS PLAIT.*

One of the biggest gluten incidents was actually at a high-end boutique restaurant that is owned by gluten-intolerant people who stress their knowledge of gluten-free dining. I know, *right*? It's like being slapped in the face by a friend.

I had been there before with Non-GFBF (before he went fully gluten free), and we grilled the server and felt very safe with our order. We were very happy with our service and especially loved that when we

87

said that we were celiac, the server knew exactly what we were talking about because his family all had celiac disease (lucky us). We loved the food, even if it was expensive ($20 an entrée, more for appetizers, and an entire paycheck for a bottle of high-priced wine).

A few months later, my girlfriends were in town on tour, and I wanted to take them out to a nice restaurant. I rarely get to see them, and I felt like a nice dinner would be perfect. The whole time we were driving to the restaurant, I talked to them about how friendly this restaurant is to specialty diets (vegetarian, vegan, gluten-free, etc.) and bragged about the place being owned by people with gluten intolerance.

I ordered the following: *pork osso buco confit, spaetzle, 18 gf.*

I have to admit that the only thing I knew in that entire mouthful was "pork." Don't judge. After I ordered the dish I asked, "That's gluten-free, right?" He replied, "Yes, everything is made fresh." Although that wasn't *quite* the reply that I was looking for—I didn't think twice about it. Why? Because I didn't have a clue what the hell *spaetzle* was. I just saw the "GF" on the menu and went for it. This is where I acknowledge that I failed in several ways: 1) I didn't know what an item was and blindly followed the description on the menu. I didn't want to be "that girl" who asks "what is that!?!?!" all loud and uncultured at a fancy restaurant. Still my fault though. 2) I didn't blatantly call out that I have a "severe food allergy" and/or that I had celiac disease. When the server replied with something that wasn't word-for-word, "Yes, that is gluten free," I should have inquired further. 3) I didn't really read that the key for GF on the menu was actually "gluten free or request gluten free." I HATE that restaurants do that. Just add an R in front of the GF for God's sake—it's just one letter, and it could have saved my ass.

When I received the plate, it looked amazing so I didn't second-guess anything. I dove in and loved everything. The vegetables were intermixed with the *spaetzle* so I grabbed a few veggies and ate a few bites of what I thought was some sort of gluten-free potato gnocchi. I knew that something was off when I ate it—it just didn't seem right. It tasted delicious, but it definitely tasted like gluten. I had never been glutened before at a restaurant, so I just kept eating without remorse. About two more forkfuls later, the wheels started turning in my head, and my Spidey Sense started tingling. The next time the waiter came back, I asked about the dish being gluten free. *It wasn't. Awesome.* He explained that he didn't understand that I needed the dish to be gluten free, and that the dish definitely was packed full of vitamin G—gluten. I was with my girlfriends, so I tried to not panic and enjoyed the rest of the plate—the pork—and get home as soon as I could.

After dropping my friends off, I drove home and immediately Googled *spaetzle*, and found out that, indeed, it was a type of German noodle dish with—you guessed it—flour. *Son of a bitch.*

Since it was my first time exposing myself to straight-up gluten since really going gluten free, I had no idea how I would react. I know from my past that I wouldn't have explosive stomach issues, but I was treading on new territory. All I could do was just wait it out and see what happened!

The next day, I woke up feeling like a brat. I was an emotional wreck, and I didn't know if it was from the gluten or from feeling like the biggest fool because I screwed up just as badly as the server did (not that bad, but I still had *some* blame). At that point, the only thing that would have made me feel better would be to call the restaurant and tell them what happened.

I called the restaurant and asked to talk to the manager. I ended up just sobbing and choking out my story. The manager was so apologetic, and was very understanding of the problem. She also informed me that it wasn't just the *spaetzle* they would have to change to make the dish really gluten free. Apparently the sauce on the pork was full of gluten too. Seriously folks, I can't make this up. The gluten-free item had more gluten in it than most meals I made at home pre-diagnosis. I eventually had to rat out the server (who apparently was going to get a strict punishment for not listening better to the customer) and was assured that it wouldn't happen to me again. My name was put on a special list, and I was assured that if I came back, I would have a free meal and that

I would be assigned the server I had before (with the celiac family and therefore a empathetic server).

We have not been back since.

THAT SASSY BITCH SOY SAUCE STRIKES AGAIN.

One of the most epic glutening experiences was also one of the most prolific yet. I organized the blogger team for the Celiac Disease Foundation national conference in Los Angeles. Along with the CDF team, I got to work with the blogger team in promoting the event and spreading the news to the public about the new info we learned in the expo. Like it wasn't enough work on my plate, I also decided that organizing a blogger dinner sounded like a good idea. I think it's totally Murphy's Law that someone would get glutened when I got 10 gluten-free people together for a dinner.

There were several restaurants on FindMeGlutenFree.com that were close to the event's venue, but none that I trusted more than PF Chang's. On a corporate level, they do the absolute best to take care of gluten-free patrons. They have a separate menu, a separate area in the back and even have designated plates for the gluten-free food. They understand cross-contamination, and they understand our issues. Personally, I've always felt so safe and so taken care of at my PF Chang's. Maybe I was just on a lucky streak.

About a month ahead I called the general manager of the restaurant and asked all of the questions I normally do when I visit a joint. He passed the test and was very excited to host a group of bloggers. The day of the event, I went in early and asked to meet with the manager to discuss the game plan (a.k.a. everything has to be gluten free—duh). It was a different manager, but this one also passed the test and assured me that his staff was excited to serve us and to keep us safe. Our waiter appeared to be well versed in the gluten-free menu, and we were very explicit when we ordered that everyone was getting gluten-free items. After we ordered, the manager even came up to us to see how everything was going. Things were looking up and I was very excited about our safe meal—and looking forward to giving PF Chang's some great publicity for hosting so many well-known bloggers.

Or not.

The majority of the meals came out perfectly fine, on the PF Chang's special gluten-free plates. Then a blogger ordered the gluten-free Shanghai Cucumbers, which are supposed to be sliced cucumbers sprinkled with soy sauce and sesame seeds. They came out and weren't on a special plate, but it was a very small side-dish order. I was sure that they had just used a small plate to bring out the small dish. But, remember what I said about assumptions. When we asked the server about why the dish was different from the other dishes, and he was puzzled too. At first, he fibbed to us (another trait I hate) and assured us that it was gluten free, but he would just check to make sure. Then, the manager approached the table. This time, he had a worried look in his eye, and I knew that the interaction would go poorly.

He informed us that the dish was not gluten free, and that there had been a mix-up in the kitchen. Seriously—*you can't make this up*. A group of influential gluten-free bloggers served gluten during a gluten-free conference. If I were the manager, I would be so devastatingly embarrassed. Luckily, he was. I don't like to wish misery upon others, but when someone messes up this badly, I don't feel bad about making them feel just as bad as we do. Granted, the manager had not screwed up the dish—he didn't sprinkle soy sauce on the dish instead of tamari. He didn't deliver the dish to the table and not confirm that it was gluten free. But, he did make me a promise, and he didn't supervise his staff enough—*clearly*.

Lucky for me, there were several other bloggers there to have my back. I was so angry—angry to the point of tears. I couldn't contain myself and instead burst into tears. I was *so* embarrassed. I kept thinking that all of the other bloggers would hate me because I brought them to this restaurant and made them sick. I thought that my readers would be disappointed in my experience and start rants online like, "This is precisely why I don't eat out ever," and start to convince others that even the best celiac can never be safe. I was disappointed and heartbroken that even when you do everything right, someone can still screw up. *Heartbroken.*

After telling the manager how angry and disappointed I was, tears started coming for a different reason. I sobbed to the manager, "This is why we are advocates, and this is what we are fighting for. We are fighting for the respect we deserve at a restaurant. We try so hard, and yet we can't even eat safe." I don't really remember everything I said because at this point I was already past the point of anxiety, past the point where logical reasoning lived, and my primal brain stepped in. I went to the bathroom and locked myself in the stall and just cried.

When I came out, it was clear that the other bloggers knew I had hit my crazy point. The manager came over, and for the next thirty minutes, apologized to me and another blogger who was trying to explain to him the severity of the situation. Yes, it was just a *little* soy sauce—but that little bit caused some pretty grotesque after-effects for the few bloggers who ate the dish. He did everything he could to make the situation better. Although he knew he couldn't ever fix it, he could try his hardest (within his realm) to make it better. While at first only those who were affected were offered gift cards, the bloggers stuck up for all of us, and we were all offered gift cards for the experience. I believe that those directly affected were contacted by the corporate office. While these actions didn't make things right, it's the best they could offer us. They also promised to continue training their staff and reporting best practices to corporate to assure that this never happened again. And we totally made him cry. I try not to be a bully, but it was pretty awesome to see that he teared up after watching me bawl like a hot mess for so long.

I still trust PF Chang's and would definitely choose them over other restaurants that don't have an extensive program to teach their staff about gluten free. However, I make sure that I watch everything like a hawk and double- and triple-check my meals there.

GLUTEN-FREE CONTAMINATED PANCAKES ARE OUR SPECIALTY.

Last October, Non-GFBF and I flew out to Denver for our friend's wedding. Yes, it's the same vacation during which I also tripped over a sidewalk and subsequently had really painful knee surgery.[29] At first, I was excited to book a trip to Denver because I had heard that it was such a gluten-free-friendly city. On the last day there, however, I was hobbling around on a full knee-brace like an asshole, and was so not stoked to be in Denver still. I just wanted to be home in bed. But we still had to eat, so we patronized a breakfast joint in Denver that specializes in pancakes, waffles and other awesome breakfast foods. I found them via a gluten-free search engine and was impressed with their online menu. I was excited to check out their pancakes, as they sounded amazing. But, I was more excited when I saw the English muffins because I'm a sucker for breakfast sandwiches.

When we sat down (after a few minutes of trying to figure out the best way to sit while wearing a giant immobilizer on my leg), I was so eager to explore all the great food I could eat.

And then I made a mistake—I asked the server how it was all prepared.

They toast the gluten-free muffins in the same toaster as gluten bread.

They make the gluten-free waffles in the same waffle maker as the gluten waffles.

They make the gluten-free pancakes on the same griddle as the gluten ones.
Seriously.

---

[29] Not that it's relevant, but the couple are no longer married. So you know, looking back it's not my *favorite* vacation I've ever had in my life.

Although my server was *so* nice, she really knew nothing about what needs to happen when dining out gluten free. When I asked her about ingredients in the syrup, she admitted *she didn't really know what gluten was*. She said that she had heard so many different ideas of what gluten was and what gluten free was from her customers. Like you needed more reasons on why the gluten-free trend hurts people who actually eat gluten free. I literally said the first thing that came out of my mouth: "Well that's scary." Again, do I need to give more examples of why this gluten-free food trend is a pain in my ass? Because of the trend, this server had heard all the wrong things about gluten free and assumed that as long as a product was gluten free, it was fine for everyone regardless of how and where it was cooked. I wanted to wring her neck and tell her to stop paying attention to those assholes who order gluten free and then sneak bites of "real" pancakes off of their friend's plate. Steam was coming out of my ears.

She went back to her manager and talked to her a little more and assured me that all the syrups but one were gluten free and that they could prepare my gluten-free pancakes in a separate and new pan that was off the griddle.

Should I have left immediately? Yes. *However,* I had just broken my knee and was on the injured reserve list with a brace. I didn't want to wobble around downtown Denver looking for another gluten-free place where I could eat. Emotionally, I just couldn't take it anymore. So, I hoped for the best and when placing my order I asked her to follow the right protocols.

After that, it seemed like the staff knew I was serious about not getting sick. I took a few minutes and explained that there were people who order gluten free because they think it's healthier, but that I had a serious condition that meant I couldn't eat anything that contained or touched gluten, and that by using the same griddle or toaster as gluten made the food not gluten-free.

I have no idea how other gluten-free people haven't complained about getting sick there. I don't know how they couldn't get sick there with the restaurant using the same toaster, etc. Then again, maybe they were just eating there to be trendy.

NEVER TRUST SOMEONE WHO CLAIMS, "OH I TOTALLY KNOW SOMEONE WITH 'CELIACS,'" AND THEN SERVES YOU GLUTEN.

My gluten-free girlfriend Mary Fran and I went to a blogging conference in Chicago. We checked with the conference in advance to see if they were able to serve us safely (multiple times). We were assured that they were used to serving gluten-free guests and that every day there would be a separate buffet labeled clearly for people like us.

During lunchtime on the first full day of the conference, regular *full-gluten rolls* were placed next to (and in the same basket with) gluten-free rolls. They were *labeled* on the gluten-free table as gluten-free rolls. See where the problem is? When we approached the table to get our lunch, our fellow gluten-free friend was already in discussion with one of the servers, as she had taken a bite of a roll. The roll she ate was *so* delicious she had to question it (isn't that a sad statement?). The server came back and told us that it was a mistake and took the whole plate of gluten and gluten-free rolls to the back-of-house. The server made it seem like once the rolls were taken into the back, everything was right again.

I flagged the staff and demanded to talk to a catering manager about this issue—as eating a whole gluten roll is a little more extreme than just the typical cross-contaminated surfaces I thought I'd have to deal with during the conference. Something like *that* could take a blogger out for weeks or months. If Mary Fran had been the unfortunate one to eat it, she would have had to inject an EpiPen into her thigh and get rushed to an emergency room. And that doesn't sound like a place I wanted to go to. The blogger who ate the gluten roll forced herself to throw up the gluten so she wouldn't be bedridden. What an *exciting* day.

We then talked to the catering sales manager and told her how serious the mistake was. She (incorrectly) said that the sick blogger just ate a white flour roll so she didn't think she would be that sick. *SERIOUSLY.*

Wrong—any gluten would make you sick as a dog, regardless of white or wheat. That type of incompetence in the food industry is alarming, and we told her that the statement alone made us afraid to eat there and afraid for everyone else to eat there. She assured me that she would talk to the chef and take care of it. The chef came out and *personally* made us a lunch and was very apologetic. We worked it out with the catering manager that all of us would come directly to her and she would have the chef specially prepare meals for us celiacs/wheat-allergy folks to assure our safety. We were satisfied with that answer, but obviously a little skeptical of the safety of the buffets for the conference.

This was an unfortunate problem with the catering team for the venue, not with the conference team, although unfortunately the two are intertwined because our meals were part of the conference ticket. What makes this whole situation much worse is that they served us gluten *again* on the second day.

We arrived at breakfast on Saturday and asked for our specialty gluten-free plates to be delivered (as per our previous instructions with the catering team). Just to be sure (because we always have to cover our butts), I went back to the supposedly "gluten free" buffet table and compared what was on that buffet table to what we were served directly from the chef. Our chef-selected plate was one-third full of seitan (which is just vegan wheat gluten, yes, gluten). Although it looked awesome, it wasn't something I wanted to eat. Once again we had to call the catering manager and express just how awful this incident was. She then brought out the banquet director who assured us that they were (once again, seriously) mistaken and that they would make us special meals. They finally brought out a plate of basically just bacon and sausage. By this point we were so frustrated and I told Mary Fran that I wanted to skip the second day of the conference because I was so emotional and frustrated that I couldn't even "learn" over my anger about the situation. *Le sigh.*

As a final note, I contacted the conference and informed them in depth about the incidents with their catering company. They assured me that they strive to be as accommodating as possible to those who need a gluten-free diet. I put my trust in them, and they have *tried* to make everything right with those who were affected by the incident. I know that this incident will only help them understand the importance of working with specialty-diet bloggers in the future for upcoming conferences. They understand the seriousness of the two incidents, and are having post-conference chats with the venue and catering teams to address the incidents.

Again, every shitty incident is an opportunity for someone to learn and for you to create change for others. I hate that we have to have negative incidents in order for people to take us seriously enough to make changes for the next person. Unfortunately, until gluten-free food and our lifestyle are taken seriously, we will be dealing with these episodes. But we're here to keep fighting the good food fight so the people who get diagnosed after us can live a life free of worry and experiences like these.

Combating a Fad Dieting Myth

A "fad" diet is something that comes and goes—something that's "so hot" right now, and then fades away. Trendy new diets appear faster than clothing trends like harem pants and scrunchies. Take it from someone who buys outfits off of vintage sale racks—I'm no trendsetter. But unfortunately I've become trendy (and so have you!) in the way that I eat. I'm all for people who want to lose weight and get in shape in a healthy manner. However, I really just wish that my diet (or should I say my *lifestyle*) wasn't one that was catching on as a trendy new way to lose weight. Trends are now making gluten out to be a weight-inducing villain, and I'm sick of feeling trendy.

Part of my job as an advocate is to "get the word out" about what a gluten-free diet is all about—from what celiac disease is to how restaurants can properly meet our needs. However, one huge roadblock always gets in the way of this advocacy, and it's all about weight loss and "healthy" eating. I'm using quotes around "healthy," because many gluten-free items are more calorically dense than their gluten counterparts. This drives me bonkers!

During the past few years, I have had to navigate conversations like this via social media about being gluten free.

"Will I lose weight on the gluten-free diet?" (*Not if you eat gluten-free donuts and pizza every night*)

"<via Instagram> Gluten-free pizza! #fitspo #healthyeating #cleaneating #fitness #healthydiet" (*Pizza is not fitness or clean eating just because it is gluten-free crust with a lb. of cheese and pepperoni*)

"I'm going to try the gluten-free diet next after I finish my juice cleanse. My yoga instructor said it totally made her chi focus." (*So I elaborated on the absurdity of this a little, but I see too many fit bloggers out there going from juice fast to gluten-free eating to paleo dieting so much that it confuses people—making them think gluten-free bread is so much healthier!*)

"How much weight have you lost since going gluten free?" (*Uh, I gained 15 pounds . . . so negative 15 lbs.?*)

I wish that "gluten free" equated to "medically necessary diet only,"[30] but that's not the case. I don't know how many times I've written that being gluten free is a lifestyle and not a diet—but I'm sick of writing it. While fad can mean "for a day," I was hoping that's how long the gluten-free trend would last. However, it looks like the trend is only gaining momentum.

Here are some stats from *New Hope Natural Media in 2013*[31] that make me question whether I should be super stoked or super disappointed.

---

[30] I also include those looking for an anti-inflammatory diet for conditions like autism and fibromyalgia into this category of "medically necessary." I want to include anyone who isn't doing this just because it's the new "it" diet and trending. I want people engaging in a 100% gluten-free diet because it's benefiting them medically, not just because they want to lose belly fat.

[31] Statistics are from NewHope360.com, including stats from Packaged Facts and the NPD Group.

+ **29%**—Americans who say they are trying to avoid gluten for health reasons
+ **#2**—Where "gluten free" was ranked in *Time* magazine's Top 10 Food Trends of 2012
+ **$4.2 billion**—The size of the 2012 US gluten-free market
+ **$6.6 billion**—The expected size of the gluten-free category by 2017

But why is gluten free the next big "it" thing? Celebrities are one part of the equation. They are latching on to the gluten-free diet like a gold-spouting wheat-free teat. Gwyneth Paltrow, Kim Kardashian, Miley Cyrus, and Lady Gaga are only a few of the stars who make my life miserable. The use of the label "gluten free" to describe their weight-loss techniques or "healthy" eating (instead of a medically prescribed diet) has run rampant. Why don't celebrities call it like it is: going Paleo (if that's the case) or going low-carb (or "low-gluten"—or what I like to call "seriously annoying") like in the case of celebrities who splurge on real cake or cookies as a treat on a gluten-free diet. If Gwyneth Paltrow lets her kids cheat with Oreos, that's not a real gluten-free diet, is it? If a celiac did that, he or she would have major ramifications.

Notice that I'm not mentioning celebrities with celiac disease because most of them are doing it right (although I've had some Twitter exchanges with those that *don't*). I don't care if you're uber famous or the girl next door—if you have celiac or NCGS and are doing everything right about your diet and advocating for it, I commend you.

But it doesn't end with dieting-obsessed celebs in the public eye. The trend continues to celebrity TV health professionals too. I swear to you, if I hear one more person saying, "The other day on Dr. Oz he was talking about gluten. . . ." Dr. Oz is like Dr. Phil and Oprah—whereas everyone who watches them automatically becomes obnoxious and a self-proclaimed doctor or therapist. I would know because I love Dr. Phil and often find myself talking back to the television when I watch an episode. And on more than one occasion my mother has told me that some condition I was complaining about was probably due to (fill-in-the-blank health disaster) she saw once on Dr. Oz.

The marketing behind celebrity doctors and therapists is just as powerful (if not more) as Hollywood actresses and can be judged by the sales of their books and by the featured products flying off the shelves.[32]

While I do respect these celebrities for bringing gluten issues to the forefront, I'm scared that too many people are following the advice of a TV doctor instead of visiting their own physician to seek the answers they need. If everyone who thought they had celiac or NCGS blindly followed advice from the television, we would have a lot of misdiagnosis out there. There's always a disclaimer to cover their ass at the end of their shows, but how many people follow that?

Are you asking yourself why I wouldn't be super stoked about all this? It's a total Catch-22 really. More manufacturers are getting on board with gluten-free products, and ultimately that means more gluten-free food for us! By going mainstream, gluten-free food will become more prevalent in the average grocery store and at restaurants. But on the flip side, many manufacturers are just trying to fulfill the latest marketing craze and aren't taking gluten-free manufacturing seriously (a.k.a., a dedicated line, a dedicated facility, ELISA testing, etc.).

As people with celiac disease, we have to fight constantly for restaurants and servers to understand that the gluten-free diet is far more than just the next weight-loss trend. It's our way of surviving life and avoiding poison to our systems. Food is our only medical prescription, but celebrities who use "gluten free" as a means to lose weight and show off their trainer-toned figures are making it hard to legitimize our very strict diet and avoid cross-contamination. These spotlight-prone individuals are out there being willy-nilly with the use of "gluten free." *It literally makes me so upset I just used the word "willy-nilly."*

---

[32] If you want to learn more about it, read the *Forbes* article from 2011 called "The Oz Effect: Medicine or Marketing?" and wonder why I get alarmed when he pushes the gluten-free "diet" with little discussion about celiac disease.

Gluten-free dieting shouldn't be *dabbling* in the lifestyle. A gluten-free diet needs to be 100% or nothing at all—for the sake of everyone who is gluten free for a medical reason. I don't think they know what harm this trend could do to the safety of those with celiac disease or NCGS. Here's why it pisses me off.

1. They are not great role models for our community

I adored the coverage that the Olympic athletes got about their struggles with gluten because it addressed their very real sensitivities and intolerances. Granted, there are athletes who go gluten free to enhance their performance and then splurge on pizza after their big race, but I'm not talking about them (and will expose them every chance I get). I'm talking about those athletes who have to pack their own snacks and lunches to everything like we do. These are the types of role models that we need—those who are overcoming the odds despite this disease, the ones who talk about their struggles before going GF. We need more Dana Vollmers and Craig Pintos out there.

And what about celebrities in the public eye that are doing gluten free right? What about those who advocate for celiac disease and a gluten-free lifestyle in the right way? We need more Jennifer Espositos, fighting to bring a medically necessary gluten-free diet and celiac disease into the mainstream, not trends.

Celebrities typically have their own staff and endless time on their hands—but regular people don't have that. We plebeians have to do all of our own cooking or rely on trained restaurant staff to do the cooking for us. Living gluten free is hard work. But I haven't heard fad dieters talk about their struggles of being gluten free and trying to survive in a wheat-filled world. New to gluten free? It's easy—even Jessica Alba did it! Right?

2. I don't want to look like a trendy jackass

I have now started saying, "I am a celiac and have severe allergies to gluten. I will be ordering a gluten-free meal because of that. A severe allergy to gluten, yes—wheat, rye and barley," instead of my typical, "I'm gluten free." Why? Because of all of these trendy dieters who just order something off of the gluten-free menu and don't care about cross-contamination and ingredients. Guess what, trendy jerks? If I order the same thing without alerting the restaurant of the very real danger I have while eating out, the restaurant might be tempted to slack off on their strictness when it comes to what the gluten-free food touches, etc. After I explain my disease to servers, their ears perk up. They listen to what I say. You know why? They've probably met people who eat gluten free to be trendy, ordering gluten-free pizza and then a full-gluten cake for dessert, which minimizes our struggles while we're eating out. Like what I mentioned in the negative dining-out scenarios: One person's lax version of eating gluten free can compromise the health of many. They've made it harder for me to stand out from the crowd of people who are doing it to lose weight or because it's the new "it" thing. Guess what? Salad has always been gluten-free!

3. I gained weight

I gained weight when I went gluten free, as do many celiacs who faced malnourishment prior to diagnosis. I gained between 10 and 15 pounds. Although I was not happy with growing out of all of my clothes, suddenly I was not anemic anymore. However, when the media stresses gluten free as a way to lose weight, it's giving people false information. Yes, if you too ate nothing but protein and vegetables and cut out all carbs and sweets except a GF cookie when you were a really good girl, you could probably shed some hefty pounds. However, when doing direct substitution—like many people who must eat gluten-free—you're faced with more calorically-dense food, and you'll put on the pounds. Do people think that gluten-free bread is something magic that contains zero calories and will make your ass shrink two sizes overnight? Apparently. I troll the interwebs for people talking about how the gluten-free diet helps you shed pounds. I correct their statement and say that mindful eating and reduced calorie consumption helps people to lose weight.

Protein-heavy gluten-free grains and seeds like quinoa and vegetables spaghetti squash and zucchini are great substitutions for pasta. But, these are also found in the Paleo diet. If you want to diet, say you're dieting. But saying you're on a gluten-free diet when you're trying to lose weight minimizes my personal struggles with the gluten-free lifestyle. And you're probably pissing off many of us who have gained weight trying to find good substitutions for our favorite foods that we can no longer eat. You know, the ones that you'll go right back to eating as soon as your "diet" is over and which we'll never get to taste again.

So why do people latch onto fad diets that celebrities and talk-show hosts pimp out? People (in general—probably not you, *right?*) want an easy way out. Some people don't want to work hard, and hard work is required to lose weight and get in shape. If you've watched any of *The Biggest Loser*, you've seen those people at the gym crying and vomiting off of a treadmill for six to eight hours a day. But some people don't want to realize that they have to eat less crap, eat more good stuff, and move way more than they currently move. They don't want to walk, run, jog, stay on that elliptical and push themselves at the gym. They want shortcuts. I mean, who wouldn't? I know I would. We're a society of people with short attention spans, and we live in a culture of immediacy. However, that can't be how we live. And the popularity of the gluten-free diet is just one of the signs of people searching for the next big shortcut and next big fad that will help them shed the pounds.

And that's where something like Olestra steps in, and people have anal leakage. Do you remember Olestra? People were willing to eat chips that contained less fat and that could cause oily poops that *may* leak out of your anus when you laugh on a date, because they couldn't just skip chips and eat something healthy instead. That's the kind of culture we live in.

But I'm not a hardass. I'm not going to tell you to stop eating all processed foods and switch to a vegan clean-eating diet—because everyone has personal choice. I believe in a diet of moderation. Eat healthy, eat as clean as you can, and you can afford to give your body (or should

I say your *brain*) rewards. But even if we decide to switch up our diet to engage in incredibly healthy behavior, or decide to eat nothing but cookies and wine for a week—we can never cheat. Any diet we are on will always have to be gluten free. We will never stop being gluten free.

I just want to be taken seriously. I want others to be taken seriously too. I can't wait until the gluten-free fad-diet fad is over and what's left over from the craze is great, safe, new food and restaurants that choose to serve it properly. I want restaurants to know that if they do things right and cater to the real gluten-free people instead of just celebrity diet chasers, they can find a new revenue stream that won't go away when the trend dies. I want the celebrities to move on to the next fad diet, and I want the celebs with celiac disease and NCGS to rise to the top and show real advocacy toward the gluten-free lifestyle.

Food Bullying: Why Do People Have to Be Assholes?

I often wonder if I would be better off and/or happier if I had found out at a very young age that I was a celiac. Perhaps my life would be easier if I never knew the taste of gluten-full food, and I was used to eating a strict GF diet starting on day one. Would it have just been easier to never know the taste of a churro or funnel cake at the state fair? What about sharing a pizza on a first date in junior high?

Then I reflect on my childhood and how difficult it was just being a nerd in advanced classes. I realized how difficult it must be to navigate the challenges of being a child and being gluten free. How do you deal with birthday parties as a kid with food allergies or celiac? How do you manage surviving living in a dorm in college when you're forced to buy into a meal plan in an unsafe cafeteria? The more I hear about the challenges of growing up gluten free, the more it made me take food bullying in general seriously.

FARE (Food Allergy Research and Education) recently put out a very moving PSA called "It's Not A Joke," stressing the struggles of kids with food allergies. There are stories of children struggling to cope with food allergy bullying (like someone smearing peanut butter on the face of a kid who has peanut allergies). Seriously f-d up, right? The thought of being bullied because you can't have a cupcake like everyone else infuriates me. Sure, there are Allermates and other allergy-awareness brands that are geared toward children and keeping them safe, but they can't stop bullying.

When you send a child to school out in the real world, you are relinquishing your control over their safety. Too often this safety is monitored by those who may not know what gluten really is, where it is hiding, and what harm it can do to a child. Luckily, it seems like allergies are getting more awareness in schools (as I've seen numerous stories about peanut-free classrooms). Perhaps the gluten-free community will one day reach that level of recognition.

On top of personal advocacy, the gluten-free community needs to step up the advocacy for our children (I mean "our" in the "we are the world" sense here). When Disney airs a show that mocks a gluten-free child and shows a bully throwing a pancake at the gluten-free child with no repercussion from adults, we need to step in.

We need to get over feeling like we're Debbie Downers and instead realize that what people see in the media is a reflection of how we are treated in real life. Being the butt of a joke in the media hurts me as much as overhearing someone in line at a restaurant say that gluten free is just a joke and a fad. It's all interrelated: how we are perceived and how we are treated.

What's so messed up is that adults are bullied too. The workplace is just an older version of a classroom, complete with bullies and people who just don't understand (and don't want to). Work lunches are a nightmare. Traveling for the company can bring on panic attacks. I've cried under my desk before, and I know I can't be the only one. If I got another sideways glance from someone when I didn't have a bite of their mandatory-celebration work-purchased birthday cake, I was going to scream.

These days it seems like having celiac disease or a food allergy means bearing the brunt of a joke as well. Whenever we as a gluten-free community strike back at those who make jokes at the expense of our lifestyle, we're told that we "can't handle a joke" or "need to stop being so sensitive." What these bullies don't get is that we can't afford to be sensitive and we can't afford to joke at our own health. While I love to laugh about the potential of pooping your pants, the very real ramifications of gluten exposure aren't something to joke about.

I consider myself quite the jokester, but when I'm told to take the stick out of my ass because I've spent time advocating for my lifestyle and my community, I want to show them what it's like to *really* have a stick in my ass. Or, maybe just have them get a colonoscopy before they turn thirty. Who's laughing now?

I know that some people will be assholes and will never change. They were probably baby assholes who grew up to be adult assholes and who will grow old and be assholes in their nursing homes. And maybe they'll get a dose of their own medicine one day when they find out that they have gluten sensitivity too (or maybe that's why they were an asshole all along?). But in the face of asshole adversity, we always have to stick up for what is right for our community. Sure, we can take a light-hearted joke now and then, but jokes can only go so far without eliciting some kind of response. We need to fight back when the joke is on us, our community, and our kids.

Bullying Within Our Community

"Seize the moment. Remember all those women on the 'Titanic' who waved off the dessert cart."
—Erma Bombeck

Just when you thought it was safe in our cozy little gluten-free group, there's the topic of food bullying within our own community.

I will preface this section with the fact that I am all for health. I acknowledge the problem that America faces with obesity and poor nutrition along with food deserts and the inability to feed Americans healthy food instead of filling hungry mouths with subsidized junk. *I get it*, I do! I try my hardest to follow a healthy diet myself.

I thought that once I went gluten free and found my community, everyone there would be so full of love and puppies and sunshine. We'd all be so happy with gluten-free life that we wouldn't feel like the kid who eats alone in the bathroom at lunch. Wrong!

Some days there is as much division inside the community as there is outside. Most of it is related to food and what we choose to put inside our bodies (even if it's all gluten-free food).

Like all "diets" or should I say "food lifestyles," there will always be those who take it to the extreme. Some rely heavily on processed foods in order to get through the day, while others have adopted a more clean, whole-foods diet. You'll find these two extremes when reading any commentary on social media. Someone is always "doing it wrong," according to someone else.

Take for example those who metaphorically crap on our parade every time a new packaged food is released to the gluten-free masses. This could be new frozen cookie dough, new bread or new crackers. Maybe a blogger just posted her favorite cupcake recipe that just happens to include (gasp) butter and (gasp) sugar. The gluten-free food police who come to our "rescue" to tell us how shitty this new food is—not because it's unsafe, but because they think they know what everyone should be eating.

Comments abound about how eating processed foods makes you fat, unhealthy, lazy, etc., and these comments make me see red. Eating gluten free is hard enough as it is—*and* I'm one of those people who thinks it's "easy" after years and years of perfecting the diet (and I still struggle every now and then). When you're telling me that I'm only going to "heal," feel "100% again" or lose weight by going paleo, primal, whole 30, vegan, corn-free, soy-free, quinoa-free, GFCF, etc. I get upset. Hey, if you have done any of them and succeeded, I am so happy for you. But when it comes to a standard diet for *everyone*, I truly believe there isn't one cookie-cutter diet.

With autoimmune diseases, it's like a bowl of Lucky Charms. One bowl could have a rainbow or a horseshoe, and another could have a pot of gold (or a cockroach, whatever). What I have and what you have are probably different, as celiac disease has too many physical and emotional manifestations to name them all. We're each very different. What I have to go through in order to heal is probably not what you have to go through to heal. For example, I didn't feel better until two years into being gluten free, and I still have numerous issues. Many of my symptoms didn't go away and they might never, and that's something I just have to be okay with. However, if you tell me that I need to quit XYZ (grains, corn, soy, chocolate, coffee, dairy, music, fun, laughter, reality TV) in order to feel better, I'm going to go ahead and say, "I'm happy that works for you," instead of saying, "Oh, is that what I've been doing wrong?"

If you've gone paleo, primal, whole 30, whole 90, all-chocolate-and-cat-farts diet, or 24/7 juicing, I'm happy for you. I'm impressed that you have the discipline for any diet that you pursue on top of being gluten free. But *please* stop being a pusher—especially if you're not a celiac or gluten-sensitive person and you're just telling me to be healthier. Sometimes I want a cookie. Sometimes I want five cookies. Sometimes I want five cookies and a glass of wine. Sometimes I want a bowl of gluten-free mac and cheese and a romantic comedy. And I'm okay with that because I'm not eating only cookies and cake at every meal.

I do believe that these people are doing it with the best of intentions. They feel great, and they want others to feel great too. They believe that the guts of celiacs need extra-special care because of the damage done, and believe that processed food does more harm than good to the healing process. I believe that they really have our health in their hearts, but they leave out the mental-health aspect of learning to live with a new and very restricted diet.

Believe me, I know of the obesity epidemic that's happening in our society. It's terrifying that our kids are facing a generation with a predicted life span that is shorter than that of their parents. I juice, I make kale chips, I watch *Weight of the Nation, Food Inc.*, and I watch obesity documentaries and TV shows like they were my crack. I understand how important a well-balanced diet is, and I think the majority of us out there do understand some key components of nutrition—especially after being diagnosed.

So help me God, if I review a cookie on my blog, I want to talk about whether or not it's *safe* for us, not have a debate that this one cookie is the reason why people have to be lifted out of their houses with cranes.

Please afford people the right to have treats within the limits they feel is right for them. I will never advocate for a diet of only packaged food, without going to farmers' markets and eating real food. No one wants that *for anyone*. I think soda is awful—and if you read the book *Salt Sugar Fat*, you will too (if you didn't already). However, I will have a ginger ale every now and then without hating myself for it. When it comes to convenience, I've been there—I've needed to subsist off of boxed food, especially when traveling for business or when I've been working late at the office (and I don't even have to balance having a crazy life with kids)! We need to give gluten-free people the leeway to make the choices they think are right for them.

I'm very sensitive to the topic of food, so when someone criticizes me for the way I eat (especially when I think I eat very healthily), I feel hurt, injured and offended. I probably need a thicker skin, but I know that I speak for the people who don't necessarily have a platform upon which to talk about this subject. I'm here to speak for the people who have had disordered eating (or hell, who just have food issues) and are sensitive to the thoughts and words of others, because we're still sensitive about how we feel about ourselves.

In my humble opinion, if you want to eat processed foods—eat them. God knows that I do. I believe in everything in moderation, and if you agree with that, right on. I will eat cupcakes. I will have chocolate. I will have wine. I will blog about the latest cereal, cookie, candy, or shelf-stable product. I drink a lot of coffee and will not be fear-bullied into stopping.

I believe that eating fruits and vegetables is essential to health. If I don't have fresh fruit or vegetables in a day, I feel like crap, and I know my body wants nutrients. But when it comes to writing about food, gluten-free bloggers and authors get a bad rap because sometimes all we seem to write about is cookies and cakes. Well, fruits and vegetables have been around since the beginning (something about Eve and an apple—it's been a hell of a long time since I went to Sunday School). Since then, there's really nothing new being done to the products to market them as gluten free because they've always been gluten free, and we know it. We get excited about new cookies and new cupcakes because we're happy to have options in the world of gluten-free products.

So raise your glass of wine and toast to your health—because no one gets out of this world alive. Celebrate the time that you have here with health and moderation, but also with unrestricted happiness.

Disordered Eating and Gluten-Free Diets: More Than Just Obsessive Label Reading?

"Your body is not a temple, it's an amusement park. Enjoy the ride."
—Anthony Bourdain, *Kitchen Confidential: Adventures in the Culinary Underbelly*

I'm going to preface this chapter with the warning that I struggled with "disordered eating"[33] and eventually sought help for my problem. I am not suggesting that my story is your story or the story of anyone else with an eating disorder. This is just my story and my struggle, and maybe someone can relate. This chapter may contain triggers for those who face similar struggles.

---

[33] I'm using the term "disordered eating" because eating disorders come in all shapes and sizes. According to the National Eating Disorder Association (NEDA), these include anorexia, binge eating disorder, bulimia, and eating disorder otherwise not specified (EDNOS) for those eating disorders that don't quite fit the typical criteria. Find more information at: http://www.nationaleatingdisorders.org/types-symptoms-eating-disorders

LOW SELF-IMAGE AND THE PROBLEM WITH POPULARITY

I'm not sure I can blame my poor body image as a young adult on what I looked like as a kid. However, I found some *pretty amazing* photos of myself taken in elementary school and junior high that remind me just how awkward of a kid I really was. I was chubby with braces and frizzy hair, and I had the tackiest fashion sense—even for someone growing up in the early 90s. Clearly, I marched to the beat of a different drummer.

However, never being the popular, pretty girl was still painful. I was always the weird, funny, chubby smart girl. During a summer school acting class, I was picked to literally play the fat girl—complete with a monologue that talked all about how much I loved pizza. *Ouch.*

In junior high, I was bussed to a special school (*yes*, in a small yellow school bus) for smart kids, which from a young age I'm sure didn't help my reputation. I was smarter than many of the popular kids, and I was pretty proud of this fact. But, the popular girls always had the best-looking friends and the best-looking boyfriends and were always so much cooler than me. I hate to admit it, but I wished I wasn't the smart kid and instead, could trade it all in for a vote on Homecoming court.

I was always the girl who managed to "do it all," leading clubs and organizations and taking on overwhelming amounts of extra-curricular activities. I was always the president of everything, but never voted "most popular." I know it sounds absolutely ridiculous for a 30-year-old woman to spout off how hurtful it was that I was never part of the cool crowd. I mean, I am a grown-ass woman, with a pretty amazing life—and yet I still couldn't let it go that I was never in the running for Homecoming Queen. But how many romantic comedies take place in just this scenario? As a culture we are obsessed with being the best, the coolest, the most popular.

Of course when looking back now, I'm pretty damn happy with how I grew up. My high-ranking test scores earned me loads of college scholarships, and I've had some pretty amazing jobs (jobs that only smart people can get). But, as a kid you don't care about *that*; you care about what brand of clothes the popular kids wear, getting invited to birthday parties, and who asks you out to school dances. Needless to say, the quarterback never asked me to prom.[34]

PERFECTIONISM IS FAR FROM A PERFECT LIFE

Ever since I was a child, I've had to be perfect. I've been a high-achiever since birth, it's been hard for me to do anything but give two hundred percent to everything and overextend myself in every possible way. I think that this was a huge trigger for my disordered eating.

If I weren't the student-council president, would any college want to accept me? If I wasn't an all-state musician, should I even bother continuing to play in orchestra? And if I didn't have a thin, amazing body—what did I have? I felt like if I wasn't the total package, I might as well have nothing. If I were thin, I'd be beautiful and finally be popular and get everything I'd ever wanted. Obviously that didn't work, probably because I was a hot mess on the inside. But my eating disorder was more about aggressive self-restraint. I was always trying to achieve a state of perfection in all aspects of my life, which is a) impossible and b) *unbearable* to live with.

> Up to 24 million people of all ages and genders suffer from an eating disorder (anorexia, bulimia and binge eating disorder) in the U.S. According to the Renfrew Center Foundation for Eating Disorders.

While I don't fit all of the criteria for anorexia, I did fit the criteria for EDNOS (eating disorder not otherwise specified). Food for me was all about control: I controlled what I put in my mouth, controlled what was considered safe, and controlled how much I ate. While that may seem like I focused a lot on food, it was more about the way I felt about *my body*. I mean, I hated food—don't get me wrong—but it was more

---

[34] However, I did make out with a member of the popular high school football team during a student-council sleepover once. Then next day, he denied that it even happened. Extra ouch!

about trying to turn my body into this perfect image of how I wanted to portray myself (and food just happened to get in the way of that).

For a few years, things definitely weren't okay. I had giant bottles of chewable Tums because my stomach was never right (I don't know; maybe it was all my anxiety or the fact that I was actually hungry). I got down to less than 110 pounds, which on my 5′6″ frame made me look sickly with tiny bird arms and thighs that didn't touch. I blacked out every time I stood up, and I was pretty weak. But mostly it was a mental exhaustion that really wore me out. Trying to strive for perfection, overextending myself, and then not eating a balanced, healthy amount of food was enough to spike my anxiety to an all-time high, and that anxiety just perpetuated the cycle.

Even after I thought I was "better," I had massive issues around food. My first few years of college were rough when it came to food and eating with others. One of the worst days happened during my freshman year of college, when I took someone I was dating out to dinner with my family. I don't think I ate more than a few bites and instead I just moved food around my plate. And then I went to the bathroom and just . . . cried.

I struggled to eat on dates, and that lasted until after I graduated. It took a long time for me to be comfortable enough with a man to eat around him. My anxiety was sky high around dates that involved food, and many times I told them that I didn't feel well enough to eat so we would just hang out without food.

While some people had concerns about me, they usually addressed it by making it a joke instead of a serious issue. People always made wisecracks about how skinny I was or how I never ate at meals. Instead of disordered eating being a joke, I wish that people met it with concern and education (I don't know, kinda like how I feel about celiac disease— right?). But, luckily for me (and believe me, I'm a rarity), things got better on their own. After my first year of college, I developed more of my own sense of self and realized what triggered my anxiety and negative self-talk cycles.

The normal BMI score for someone my height would put me at 120 lbs. And I struggled when I hit that number. Getting labeled with the term "normal" was like saying I was morbidly obese. Because if I was normal, I couldn't be perfect, could I? Always being underweight gave me some sort of sick pride. But it was something I was slowly getting used to. Eventually, it started to seem weird to see pictures of my underweight self, instead of my image in the mirror at my current weight.

For a few years, things were going really well. But when I was diagnosed with gastroparesis, and then subsequently celiac disease, I was terrified that I would relapse into negative associations with food—and I think part of me did. After years of restricting my eating, I had finally healed and felt like I could eat whatever I wanted. But with this new diagnosis, I would have to focus on food even more—reading every ingredient label, asking questions about my food, and getting more anxious about eating then I ever had before.

I sought out counseling for my disordered relationship with food—finally. I was terrified of becoming "sick" again. I didn't want to be terrified of everything I ate to the point where I just wouldn't eat, or had two "safe" foods. I didn't want to spend my whole life obsessing over food. It wasn't fair to me, and it wasn't fair to my body.

I would try my hardest to avoid negative food associations and to not become preoccupied with food. I don't want to hate food. I don't want to be too terrified to give my body what it needs. I wanted to live my life enjoying what I ate and appreciate fueling my body.

WHICH CAME FIRST: CELIAC OR EDNOS?

There's not a ton of research out there on the correlation between eating disorders and celiac disease.[35] Dr. Daniel Leffler from the Celiac Center at Beth Israel Deaconess Medical Center found that over a

---

[35] Most articles I could find reference a 2007 study from the Beth Israel Deaconess Medical Center and Dr. Daniel Leffler found in the *European Journal of Gastroenterology & Hepatology*.

five-year period, 2.3 percent of the female patients they treated either had celiac disease *and* an eating disorder, or they had celiac disease that was *masquerading* as an eating disorder.

From National Foundation for Celiac Awareness' 2013 post *Celiac Disease and Eating Disorders*, author Amy Jones wrote the following:

> *"According to Dr. Leffler (personal communication, February 26, 2013): 'Celiac disease can exacerbate, precipitate or otherwise complicate eating disorders. Healthcare providers specializing in eating disorders should keep celiac disease in mind, especially if their patients have a history or family history of autoimmune diseases.'"*

I'm not sure I'm ready to make the leap that celiac disease caused my eating disorder, and I'm pretty sure it didn't. However, I know that there is a strong correlation between celiac disease and issues like anxiety and OCD, and a strong correlation between anxiety, OCD and eating disorders. So, although I won't put this in the celiac "win" column, I definitely think the two are connected—especially after I was diagnosed with celiac. All of the old feelings came rushing back about limiting my "safe" foods, and I was back to thinking about food 24/7.

I've been very lucky that I haven't relapsed when it comes to the way I eat. I *do* eat cookies and a list of unhealthy, fattening foods, but I try to regulate some of the inner guilt that comes from my old ways. I still catch myself staring at my body in the mirror and feeling disappointed. Why couldn't I lose my gut? Why do my thighs touch? As I write this, I'm at the heaviest I've ever been. I struggle with positive body image regularly—even though I believe I *am* a pretty good-looking gal. But so what if I'm not perfect, right?

I really push myself to limit negative self-talk and to try to build up others—regardless of what they look like, how much they weigh, etc. I truly believe that everyone is beautiful and everyone has something to offer the universe, even if they don't feel like it—hell, even if I don't feel like it.

But, after I became a blogger, I realized that there are people out there who want to force their diets upon others. I guess because of what I went through, I'm really sensitive to it. It angers me when someone gives me shit about posting a cookie recipe, or tells me that the only way to really feel good is to go paleo and that I'm treating my body like shit. Right now, I'm happy I'm eating in front of someone. I'm happy I have a varied diet. I'm happy I can eat that cookie without crying or spending two hours in the gym in shame or staring at my body and wondering where that cookie went. I am proud of what I'm eating and how I'm treating my body. I believe in everything in moderation because moderation is what I've always strived for. Moderation is what I never had. Moderation is way better than restrictions and extreme dieting. Moderation to me is *happiness*.

Do I want you guys to eat nothing but cookies and celebrate in the fact that you can do so? *No.* I sit up at night and read all the books about the food industry and modern-day diets, etc. I still think fast food is awful, and it's been scientifically proven to be bad for you. Do I think that it's okay in moderation? Yes, but good luck finding really good gluten-free fast food! I believe in eating as healthily as possible, including fresh fruits and vegetables at every meal and limiting carbohydrates and increasing protein. But I think that *mental health* is important to your diet too. Again, this does not mean that I think you can cheat on your gluten-free diet (because as you know, I don't believe in cheating) as your diet will make your life easier and stop your anxiety around food—but please don't take celiac as a way to hate food. I've been there too often, and I'd hate for you to be there too.

I don't do well with people telling me what to eat. It makes me feel so ashamed, like what I'm doing isn't right. I even had a nurse make some snide comment about how I should stop eating gluten-free pizza. *Thanks for that one.*

On some of these detrimental fit-spo (Fit-spiration, like fitness and inspiration had an annoying baby—clever, right? and thin-spo (the evil twin of Fitspiration) sites, I've seen the quote "nothing tastes as good as skinny feels." Well, they're wrong. Here are some examples of things that are better than being "skinny":

1. a donut
2. a piece of chocolate cake
3. a pizza

But I think it's important that everyone—not just those who are struggling with disordered eating or body image issues—realizes the difference between truth and reality.

THE MEDIA IDEA OF BEAUTY SUCKS

Those perfect images in the media are all a farce. Little girls play with Barbie dolls and idolize pop stars who hire personal trainers and have way too much time on their hands. They look at fashion models in magazines and have this false sense of reality that maybe that's how they're supposed to look. *Those* people are models for a reason. They are like one percent of the population, and let's face it—they look miserable all the time. *They* are not the average woman, and not the "average" image of beauty. Celebrities who bounce back from weight gained during pregnancy in one day have personal trainers and time on their hands. Those girls in the magazines? They are photoshopped. Barbie isn't real either—and if she was, she'd be terrifying. I'd punch real-life Barbie in the boob (because it would be at my 5′ 6″ face height) and run away screaming as if I'd just seen Godzilla. And the same goes for boys, growing up with an image of Ken, GI Joe, or Jesus—even Channing Tatum. These are unrealistic expectations for the average male, and quite frankly, it sucks to try to live up to that.

These portrayals of women are not real. Holding yourself up to that expectation is not real either. You are a real person. And real people aren't perfect. Live your life that way.

Since I've put the past behind me and sought help from professionals, I've tried to stay informed on research from NEDA and to promote healthy eating habits (including *actually* eating), healthy body image, and healthy mental state. I try not to let the number on the scale determine how I feel about myself—and neither should you.

Eating gluten-free is hard enough as it is without putting selfish restrictions and negative food associations into the mix. If you're struggling, please seek help. Please try to find a happy association with nourishing your body and learn to love the skin you are in. It may be a slow process, but it is so worth it.[36]

---

[36] Additional resources can be found at The Body Positive at thebodypositive.org and the National Eating Disorders Association at nationaleatingdisorders.org.

Dating Gluten Free:
Finding the Wheatless Man
or Woman of Your Dreams

"All you need is love.
But a little chocolate now and then doesn't hurt."
—Charles M. Schulz

While I've been gluten free for a few years now, I was single for much longer than that. And I was *really* good at being single. I did everything on my own, and I didn't need to worry about other people's preferences or agendas getting in the way of my life. It was a selfish way of living, but I had perfected it. But, at times it was also pretty lonely. While I wanted to find a mate, nothing ever really clicked with anyone. I was one hundred percent sure that I was going to be the Crazy Cat Lady from the Simpsons—alone, scaring neighborhood children, possibly eaten by felines.

I feel like a lot of people out there can relate, as not everyone can be in a healthy, committed relationship—before *or after* diagnosis. Some of us were stuck on Match.com and OkCupid hoping for the next best thing to appear in our inbox. But, after many years of looking, I finally found someone who appears to be a perfect match. But let's not spoil the ending to this chapter.

Like many other single people, I believed that dating was the absolute worst, yet necessary, part of singledom. And I'm not talking about dating without gluten: *any* dating was the bane of my existence. I promise you, I'm awful on dates. I always say the absolute wrong thing. I'm always awkward, and have even perfected the awkward robot move in any and all situations.

Dating before going gluten free was at least a bit easier. On blind dates or Match.com meet-ups I could go to any restaurant and order something tasty to share over that awkward first meal. Then together we could struggle over lulls in the conversation, but at least I didn't have to have 30 minute conversations about food with a stranger. Dating was hard for me without adding any dietary restrictions!

When I first starting eating gluten free, before I was 100% confirmed as a celiac, dating became an anxiety-provoking activity. I had to worry about: 1) eating safely; 2) not scaring off my date by talking about medical jargon and body functions; 3) not being an overall awkward human being; and 4) trying to make a connection with a stranger. It was exhausting. At times, I was happy just to stay at home for weeks and avoid human contact *just in case* I found someone and would have to go on a legitimate date.

When I met Dude #1, I sheepishly talked about my issues, and talked about going gluten free and all of my other health oddities at the time (because talking about gallbladders is sexy!). He seemed really supportive, and we went forward with trying to date like normal people. I knew that most alcohol was safe, so at first the bars were a safe place to go. After exploring local restaurants, I had a handful that I thought were safe—at least four or five places that I could go to where I could eat without having to ask the waitress a million questions.

I struggled with coming off as too aggressive when dating, because I always had to choose the restaurant ahead of time—it was never my date's job. He could never "surprise" me with a date; we had to plan on when and where we were going to eat. *Kind of a buzzkill.* He struggled to understand exactly how I needed to eat (mostly because I too was a little unsure of how to eat at the time).

During the course of our short relationship, I think we went on just two restaurant dates. Every other date, we would just hang out because it was too difficult to deal with finding a restaurant. I resigned to just eating on my own before our dates. We tried not to make food (or my health) a big portion of our time together—even though it was unmistakably a big part of my life.

Even after some time being gluten free, I still struggled with others eating gluten in front of me—especially him drinking my (formerly) favorite beer. It was too early in my diagnosis for me to be secure with my new lifestyle.

At that time, I wasn't sure how I wanted to handle gluten-free eating with a potential life partner. I didn't think that my potential life partner was required to go gluten free for my sake. I mean, c'mon, that would just make life too easy, wouldn't it?

While I am anti-food-allergy bullying (I mean, who isn't—except for the assholes who are bullying), I don't think that the entire world should be gluten free just because I am. This opinion also extends to potential life partners.

Now, I have a huge problem with the way that we've changed our food and the GMO revolution. I hate that we've changed our wheat so much since the 1950s that many of us can no longer tolerate it. Do I discourage people I know and love to think about buying non-GMO products? *Of course.* I believe in eating as naturally as possible without mentally exhausting yourself and hating yourself for having some cookies. But do I want everyone I know and love to become an anti-wheat activist? No. If you are not celiac or gluten sensitive, you are allowed to eat wheat. Go ahead!

When it comes to dating, it's less about the actual diet, and more of a matter of respect and admiration. I hope that if potential mates love me enough, they would be aware of what gluten they were eating in front of me (for example, my favorite pizza or a pink frosted donut). I wouldn't go into anaphylaxis, thankfully, if a dude ate that around me, but I would get *really sad*.

So while I had no legitimate problem with this dude drinking beer, I still don't think it was the most compassionate choice for him to make. It was really hard to deal with, especially early in my diagnosis. Needless to say, the relationship didn't work out—not just because of the gluten, but I think that was a part of it.

It really wasn't him; it was *me*.

In general, my early relationships mirrored my early gluten-free years. It was early in my gluten-free life and diagnosis, and I was too timid, too afraid, and didn't feel like myself. My early years were confusing and filled with emotional struggle and a lack of education on my end. I couldn't approach waitresses, restaurant staff and chefs like I do now. I don't think I could even truly explain it to people I cared about either!

I couldn't tell him how badly it bothered me to see him eating and drinking all of the things that I couldn't. If I wasn't sure with myself and where I was in my diagnosis, how could I be sure of any relationship or what I wanted out of someone else?

Back in the olden days, I just assumed that everything was gluten free and cross-contamination didn't exist. I didn't take the reins on my own health, because I was afraid of standing out and looking like a fool by demanding food that was not going to poison me. I was afraid of asking questions, and afraid to question anything anyone said about their food. How ridiculous.

I went through several relationships after that, and every time I was stronger in my gluten-free convictions and more set in my ways. I started going to Mayo Clinic and felt more informed than I had ever been, even on dates.

Instead of just brushing off my diagnosis as something annoying that my date shouldn't have to deal with—I shared, I educated, I informed. I was passionate about education, and mostly I was passionate about keeping myself from getting sick.

I was finally in charge of my health and I didn't let dating get in the way! I started off my introductions with phrases like, "I'm a celiac—that means I eat gluten free. No wheat, rye, or barley. No, it's not that bad, there are plenty of places for us to eat!"

I began to feel confident again, and realized that someone who was going to love me was going to love me *for all of me*—even the weird food and the cookies that always crumbled because they had no elasticity.

But, alas, several relationships ended, as I'm just terrible at dating (but apparently I'm now really good at asking if fries are cooked in the same fryer as chicken nuggets).

After a while I was beginning to think that I was going to be alone in my lifelong autoimmune disease, and thought seriously about adopting a few cats. I listened to Katy Perry's *Teenage Dream* for the first time at the gym, and by the end of the song I was filled with such singledom rage that I wanted to punch all happy-looking gym couples in the face (seriously who goes on dates to the gym?).

But then I met him—my Non-GFBF. Luckily we met as friends, so all of the awkwardness and façade of normalcy that everyone puts on during dating was out the window. When the opportunity came along, and he was freshly single, I pounced. I came in with the confidence of a champion and laid the wooing on thick. After our first few dates at gluten-free-friendly restaurants, we started legitimately dating, and I realized something awesome about this one. He genuinely, 100%, cared about my health, my diet, and everything about gluten free.

He was respectful, he was considerate, and he was kind. He praised me for doing something that "normal" people think is so tough—giving up all the great things we eat and subbing them for . . . ahem, more interesting versions of the products.

He began to eat only gluten free when we went out for dinner. He started to go shopping with me to natural marketplaces and to prepare meals together that we both could eat. He learned how to bake gluten free, and even surprised me after a long flight home with a GF pizza at the airport that he had made from scratch.

I had never found anyone who was so willing to sacrifice his own gluten happiness for a relationship. Two years later, we're still going strong and now live together in a 100% gluten-free household—even the cats have gone gluten free!

He also did something that I didn't even ask for: he stopped eating gluten. Even when I'm out of town and I tell him that he can cheat (on gluten, not on *me* obviously), he doesn't. Granted, he is a phenomenal athlete (he is a cyclist slash mountain biker slash collector of expensive bicycles and jerseys) so it's not uncommon for someone like him to give up gluten when he's training. But he does it without complaining (ninety-nine percent of the time—the other day he really wanted Denny's pancakes for some reason). While he acts 99% like a celiac—he's 100% amazing. It is truly more than I could have asked for.

I am so lucky to have someone who puts up with everything it means to be a celiac: restricted diet, crazy anxiety, expensive groceries, crowded expos and strange restaurants. His momma should be very proud.

Is this rant about my lucky situation meant to be braggadocio? No, it was meant to inspire all of you celiacs and gluten-sensitives who are currently single: know that someone is out there for you too. Believe me, I had to wait for a *very* long time and make my way through many dudes before I found the one that fit just right.

You *can* find someone who's willing to embrace your special trait and celebrate it *with you*, not make you feel timid and afraid to *be you* (and healthy)! Not all your potential mates are going to go gluten free for you (can you blame them?), but you will find someone who will be respectful of your diet and follow rules to make sure that you're not sick.[37]

If you find yourself in a relationship with someone who is not respectful or understanding of your needs, please don't accept that. It's just food—right? While dining out and social occasions around food are a large part of our social fabric, shared meals are such a small part of *love*.

---

[37] Unless you want to visit a gluten-free dating site where everyone eats like you do! When this book was published, GlutenFreeSingles.com launched and started offering a gluten-free online dating portal.

It reminds me of *When Harry Met Sally*, one of my favorite movies. Harry falls for Sally even though she is a unique individual (yes, I always thought I was a lot like Sally).

> *"I love that you get cold when it's 71 degrees out. I love that it takes you an hour and a half to order a sandwich. I love that you get a little crinkle above your nose when you're looking at me like I'm nuts. I love that after I spend the day with you, I can still smell your perfume on my clothes. And I love that you are the last person I want to talk to before I go to sleep at night. And it's not because I'm lonely, and it's not because it's New Year's Eve. I came here tonight because when you realize you want to spend the rest of your life with somebody, you want the rest of your life to start as soon as possible."*

There is someone for everyone. It's just a matter of time and effort to find them.

When you find that special someone, remember to be as respectful to him or her as they were to you. Honor their feelings and give them some slack and understanding as they adjust to being with someone with food issues. Show them love and support through their own struggles. Everyone has issues—and sometimes celiac overwhelms our world. Sometimes celiac disease and being gluten free is all I can think about. We can't let gluten free run our relationships and take center stage in our lives. It's not fair to us, and it's not fair to our partners. Let a gluten-free and safe lifestyle be an important part of your life together, but remember to nurture your relationship too!

Gluten-Free Family and Events: How to Not Stab a Family Member at Thanksgiving

"It seems to me that our three basic needs, for food and security and love, are so mixed and mingled and entwined that we cannot straightly think of one without the others."
—M. F. K. Fisher, *The Art of Eating*

Holidays are always rough. There's really no other time when we are expected to bond with others *over food*. Sure, there are birthdays and family dinners, but usually those involve very small groups or are dedicated to *you*—so there's less chance that you'll feel embarrassed, alone, lonely, and like a total freak who can't eat anything. Thanksgiving and Christmas—especially—are all about food. On turkey day, we're thankful for our friends and family—and thankful that we have food on our table and that we can share it with others. That day we're thankful for endless pumpkin pie and Pepto Bismol. With Christmas, 'tis the season for sharing homemade treats and goodies from "Santa," and lots of snacking while opening gifts. It's the time for fruitcake, bread pudding, and sugar cookies that are shaped like trees. Even Hanukkah Harry brings some type of *kugel* and *rugelach*.

However, with people like *us*, the above-mentioned goodies are enough to make us gag and cry into our bedazzled holiday stocking. Since we can't often share in many holiday dishes (unless you have a strictly gluten-free holiday, free of cross-contamination), preparing and eating your own dinner can make you feel isolated. But, we can't think about it that way.

We should use this day—like all days—as a day of feeling awesome about our bodies and being an advocate for safe, gluten-free eating.

Some of you are lucky enough to have very small family meals for the holidays. I, however, have a massive extended family. Maybe it's just because I am an only child, but having that many people in my house is overwhelming, even without bringing food into the picture. Lucky for us, we drink a *lot* of wine during the holidays to ease the anxiety.

Since I've managed not to stab a family member during a major holiday since my diagnosis, I've decided to share some tips with you that will help you manage your festivities.

Be Open About Your Food Allergies
+ Explain that you want to share this holiday with your family, but you don't want to get sick and ruin the fun for everyone. Explain how severe celiac or gluten sensitivity is—even a crumb can make you ill (and people tend to get that analogy more than rattling off the science of 20 ppm).
+ You don't need to stand on top of the table and announce to the entire family that you are eating off of your own menu. If you are more soft-spoken than I am, feel free to address family members one on one. Or, address them only when you are questioned why you're not eating grandma's stuffing. Gluten does not have to be the star of your holiday if you don't want it to be.

Bring and Cook Your Own Food
+ If traveling by car, take along a few favorite gluten-free dishes. This ensures that you will have safe foods to enjoy, even if

there isn't another dish available at your destination that you can eat.

+ It's obviously easiest to bring food that is already cooked and prepared. You won't have to deal with any unfamiliar surfaces and second-guess all of your relatives who assure you "don't worry, it's clean!"

+ If you absolutely have to cook your own food, take charge in the kitchen. Ask the mother hen (the person who rules the kitchen and is probably supervising the entire holiday cooking process—a.k.a. my mother), when and how you can prepare your item. Make sure that you sanitize everything. I know that my mom hates when I rewash every dish, utensil and surface at their house, but sometimes it's easier to be safe than riddled with anxiety. Sanitize everything and do without wooden carving boards and utensils.

Don't Be Afraid to Bake

+ There are so many gluten-free holiday recipes available online through recipe sites and gluten-free blogs. Google to your heart's content! Go nuts on Pinterest! I have faith that you can find a recipe that will work for your holiday gathering, keep you safe, and delight the taste buds of your family and friends. If the recipes seem too overwhelming, visit your local Whole Foods for plenty of boxed mixes or starter kits.

+ While you should face your fears, make sure you have the right expectations for your baking. I am known to be kitchen impaired, but for some reason I thought I would be Martha Stewart as soon as I went gluten free. Yeah, unfortunately just waking up one day and becoming a master baker is not a perk of this disease. I cut out recipes from *Real Simple* and scoured the Internet for a pumpkin pie recipe that seemed conquerable. I ended up making it and got ridiculed by everyone there (including my parents) because it looked so awful. It was literally one of the worst things I've made to-date. I kept the picture because one day, if I ever become a trained culinary expert, I will get a chance to look back at that failure and laugh. I don't even think it tasted that great, and it took every ounce of strength in my body to make it the night before (and by "night before" I mean I was seriously up until 1 a.m. making it). I would have done better purchasing the pie from a gluten-free bakery or just showing up with a bottle of vodka.

If You're Not Sure—Don't Eat It!

✦ There's nothing quite as ironic (or should I say "shitty timing") as being sick over the holidays during key vacation time. It's better to stick only to the food that you know (which is typically the food that you made), and don't eat something just because your aunt says, "I think it's gluten free." Trust me, it's not worth it.

You've Gotta Keep It Separated

✦ Designate a separate table for gluten-free items—complete with separate serving ware. You can even individually wrap cookies and slices of cake/pie so you can have single servings without the threat of contamination. Consider gluten-free stickers and labels (Allermates, Kemnitz Family, Gluten Free Labels).

I'm Totally Okay With You Hosting a 100% Gluten-Free Holiday

✦ Some people may disagree with me on this one, but I give you permission to not allow any gluten inside your home if you are hosting a holiday gathering. It's just as easy for you to ask guests to bring nonfood items such as decorations, plates and napkins, alcohol, approved side dishes (like packaged food by trusted manufacturers) and naturally gluten-free food items (like natural cheese, milk, vegetables—without shady dip—fruit bowls, etc.).

✦ While this may work on paper, I'm sure someone is going to forget or rebel and bring a gluten-filled "gift." If that happened to me, I would probably fly off the handle and scream at them about reading their Evite—but what kind of holiday cheer would that bring? Accept it graciously and if you must serve it, serve it *away* from other foods to prevent cross-contamination. We always have a separate table for GF items, or, if you're hosting, put separate serving stuff at a table by itself and make sure you label *everything* gluten.

Go Crazy at the Grocery Store

Some helpful things that I always keep on hand for large holiday gatherings:

✦ Gluten-free gravy. Imagine Foods has a boxed version of gravy, but there are numerous others on the market. You really can't tell the difference—if you have a choice, make all the gravy gluten free. If you like to make it from scratch, just use gluten-free flour blends instead of regular flour to mix with the turkey juices.

✦ Jellied cranberry sauce. Not that regular cranberry sauce is nothing more than cranberry puree, but when people bring over cranberry items they always add the strangest things to them. Marshmallows? Why?

✦ Gluten-free stuffing. I order mine online from the local gluten-free bakery, but you can make your own using dried gluten-free bread, or buy kits in the store.

✦ Easy holiday-themed mixes like Simply Organic gluten-free pumpkin cake mix or Wholesome Chow spice cake mixes. Sugar = yummy.

Easy Gluten Holiday Mistakes

There are several things I tend to forget about over the holidays, and every year I swear that I won't forget about them for next year: These things might get you glutened if you're not paying attention.

+ Make sure the people cooking the turkey don't use flour in the bag. Many bags require that you sprinkle flour to coat the bag, so make sure you get gluten-free flour before the turkey is even in the oven! Also, be wary of prebasted or self-basting turkey. The basting could hide potential glutens! Offer to pitch in on buying a GF turkey in order to feel safe without being a "complainer" or a "worry wart." Gluten-free honey-baked ham is also a great alternative meat product for the holidays.

+ Watch out for those awesome green bean casseroles—they are made with fried onions and cream of mushroom soup (often both are full of gluten). You can buy your own cream soups (brands like Pacific Foods or Imagine Foods) at natural food stores such as Whole Foods. There are also plenty of French-fried gluten-free onion recipes online too! It's all about recreating your holiday favorites in a safe way.

Other Potentially Awkward Holiday Celebrations

I feel like I'm a pro at family gatherings now. I make all my own safe food, set it up in a little safe area, and use safe utensils. I feel so, well, *safe*. I know nothing is going to get me sick because I made it all myself. I witnessed every step in the cooking and plating process. I can lecture a group of people about not touching my stuff with dirty hands/forks, etc., because they are *my* family. They are genetically predisposed to love me, even if I'm annoying (I don't know why I bothered writing "if"). However, it's a little difficult for me to go past the realm of family gatherings and move to celebrations outside the familiar—from meeting the in-laws for Thanksgiving dinner, to a New Year's Eve party to a Passover *seder* full of old ladies for whom I secretly want to learn Yiddish.

Let's take my experience at synagogue, because who doesn't love a story that could potentially end in me attempting to read Hebrew even though I never had a *bat mitzvah*. At the annual women's seder, everyone brings in some homemade kosher goodies and sets them on a long buffet line. Little gluten-free sticky notes announcing each dish's celiac-friendly nature and their need for separate utensils complemented my items. But that's for *my* food—what about everything else?

I guess I could stand up, announce my condition to the congregation, and lecture them about not touching my stuff and alerting me of any potential allergens or cross-contamination in their dishes, but instead I sat quietly and chose not to eat. I ate a few things that I know are GF—like fresh-cut bell pepper, hard-boiled eggs, and my food—but that's it. Although a lady next to me said that her *kugel* (I know I'm a terrible half-Jew but I still spelled that right the first time) was gluten free, I didn't have the time or patience to delve into it with her. How did you make it? Fresh utensils? A clean surface? Are you sure your ingredients are sourced properly? What about sauces? You know the drill . . . I just didn't try it. There was a lady at my table who was gluten free, but she only did so because she believes it is healthier for her. I envied her because she could trust everyone who said their dish was gluten free. However, I don't want to risk another ulcer or impaired mental clarity because I want to "fit in." I did want to believe the sweet lady who made *kugel*—*I did*—but my intestines make me question everyone. *Oy vey.*

Another potentially awkward situation was my first dinner with the dude's parents. While they knew I was gluten free, they (like anyone) didn't know to what lengths I had to go in order to avoid getting sick. Then again, *I* didn't really know to what lengths I had to go in order to avoid getting sick. In fact, I helped make "gluten free" no-bake cookies with his mom, using traditional Quaker (aka contaminated) oatmeal. No wonder I was getting sick when I went there!

I was embarrassed to explain to my pseudo in-laws about how I had to be so careful when preparing my food at someone else's house. I was afraid that they'd think I wasn't good enough for their son because I was some creepy food weirdo. I mean *I know* that Non-GFBF is eating better than before, and we're both more cognizant of the food we're putting into our bodies. But still, I want others to know that he's not living a subpar life just because he's chosen to give up gluten for me.

Thankfully, his parents are supportive of his change and are very supportive of us and the website. I really think they are as proud of their son for designing some kick-ass awareness shirts as I am!

Gluten-Free Holiday Fun

But let's not make *all* holidays and events seem depressing. Holidays can also be an opportunity for celiac awareness. Take Halloween for example.

Halloween is probably my favorite holiday next to Christmas. I love the concept of being someone else and dressing up with lots of props. I guess that's the former theater geek in me. Since I'm all about advocacy, let's talk about creative Halloween ideas for those with celiac or NCGS. Get your hot-glue gun out because these are going to take some work.

+ **Scary stalk of wheat:** Go to Michaels or Hobby Lobby and buy several stalks of fake wheat. Take your bedazzled hot-glue gun (oh c'mon, you have that too, right?) and glue the bottom of the stalks to a white t-shirt. Buy a set of vampire fangs and some fake blood. Buy a black cape. Go around to trick-or-treaters saying "I want to steal your nutrients!" I know I'd be scared.

+ **Wheat Belly:** Carry a copy of *Wheat Belly* by William Davis around and stuff an oversized shirt with pillows to create the appearance of a large inflamed belly. Bonus points if you wear their t-shirt. Yes, apparently they even sell a Wheat Belly t-shirt. It's a marketing machine, I tell ya.

+ **Zombie Celiac:** Go as yourself but in zombie make-up (à la *The Walking Dead*). Tell everyone that you've been living in a zombie-like haze because the restaurant you love actually prepares its food in an unsafe, cross-contaminated environment. Bonus if you give yourself mouth ulcers and lose ten pounds to make it seem more real (but seriously, don't do that).

+ **Doctor who understands:** Wear scrubs and latex gloves. Pass out fake Rx for a gluten-free diet, IgA tests, genetic tests, or endoscopies. Bonus points if you can actually score Mayo Clinic scrubs. Extra special bonus points if you actually advocate hard enough that someone gets tested for celiac disease!

+ **Elisabeth Hasselbeck:** Dress adorable, act incredibly perky, carry a coffee cup that has *The View* logo on one side and the Fox News logo on the other, and a copy of her *GFree Diet* book. Be overly positive and talk people's ear off about how a gluten-free diet makes you feel 100% better, even if you don't *need* to be on it.

+ **Obsessed Paleo Dieter:** Literally dress like a caveman. Carry around a giant turkey leg like you find at the fair. Slap all of the candy and chocolate out of the hands of people, and give them Ziploc bags of fresh vegetables instead.

+ **Gluten Free Gordon Ramsey:** Dress in a white chef's coat and have a hefty British accent and swear constantly (not safe for a children's costume or a children's party FYI). Go on and on about how restaurants that have gluten-free menus, but don't understand cross-contamination, are disgusting and vile.

+ **Celiac and the Beast:** Wear your "No Wheat No Rye No Barley Gluten Free" shirt out with a pair of jeans, and ask everyone that you meet if you can review their product and blog about it. Mandatory stops at every gluten-free support group. Bonus points if you carry around a MacBook, iPhone, and a handful of KIND bars.

The overall rule of thumb with these holiday gatherings is that if you choose not to speak up, not to ask questions, not to make a fuss—you're relegated to eating nothing or suffering the potential consequences. Always put your health first. Holidays are for celebrating those who are important to us. This should bring us together and teach us to love each other for who we are and not what we eat. Keep the drama to what new tattooed dude your cousin brought to dinner, not about gluten.

Navigating Shopping—
To the Grocery Store and Beyond

I'm not sure there's anything more overwhelming than your first trip to the grocery store after being handed a gluten-free diagnosis. I remember just staring at the aisles of food—like I was discovering words for the first time and trying to put it all together in my head. I was spending hours reading every package, trying to make sense of it all. I felt like I needed an interpreter to understand some of the packaging and ingredients. Was this safe? I don't know! AHHHHHH! (Screams, pulls hair, runs out of store)

To ease your anxiety in the beginning (or just on a really difficult day or when going to a new store), stick to naturally gluten-free food found in the outside perimeter of the store. This includes unaltered fruit and vegetables, meat products, and dairy (if you're lucky enough for your stomach to handle it).

When first diagnosed, consider purchasing a grocery guide (Cecelia's Marketplace and Triumph Dining are two brands of guides) to help you navigate the store. These guides are sorted by brand and by product type. Again, things I wish I knew about when I was first diagnosed.

Some stores (Trader Joe's, Sprouts and Whole Foods for me locally) have a gluten-free product list available to help you navigate the store. If you're still having problems navigating gluten-free products, ask for help from an employee!

One of my biggest pet peeves is that the grocery stores do not have a standard location for gluten-free packaged goods. Wouldn't that make shopping so much easier? Some put the gluten-free items on a special shelf with a gluten-free sign pointing the way like the Star of Bethlehem. Some tend to aggregate gluten-free food with the "healthy food" (this really grinds my gears), along with vegan and allergen-friendly foods. The problem with this layout is that the GF food is next to the *supposedly* healthier ancient grains like spelt and kamut (or even worse, whole-wheat versions of items) and can be super confusing to navigate. Then, there are stores that fully integrate the gluten-free products with the "normal" products. And then there's Whole Foods, where things are all over the place (I think that's a tactic to get you to wander the aisles and spend more money). I really wish that the National Grocers Association would come up with a standard for where the hell I can find my gluten-free crackers.

While there are strictly gluten-free brands that are typically found in the "gluten-free only" section, mainstream brands like Chex are found amongst its gluten-full peers. And food that is typically gluten free like spaghetti sauce is found in the spaghetti sauce section with brands that are labeled GF and those that are not.

Be careful of bulk bins full of products. Although the product inside might be gluten free, you can't guarantee the cleanliness of the bin or scoop. The deli section is another scary place. Luckily for me, my grocery store offers gluten-free meat brands like Applegate in pre-packaged packs. If you're going to use the deli machine to slice fresh meat, use caution. Some meats are certified gluten free, but the deli uses the same slicer for everything. You can ask the team member to sanitize the machine before slicing your product. Just go during off-hours, so you're not holding up the deli line. The pre-made food section is one of the other areas I don't frequently visit. I just can't trust their procedures and their product knowledge of all of the ingredients used in the food. Plus, everything is far too close to that wonderful-smelling fried chicken for me to leave happy anyway. Again, it's better safe than sorry—even when you're out shopping.

I try to avoid anxiety attacks at all possible costs. Not having enough safe food in the house and not knowing what to make for dinner are two things that can shoot my anxiety levels through the roof. I try to be as prepared as possible in the kitchen to avoid staring into my cabinets and refrigerator for what seems to be hours at a time, wondering what the hell I can eat.

While many bloggers prepare an entire week's worth of meals over the weekend, let's face it—I'm just too lazy for that. I honestly have no idea how they manage to have children and manage meal prep. I'm sorry, my DVR is way too full of reality TV for that nonsense. Although I like being prepared, sometimes I do like some wiggle-room for what I'm having for dinner. So instead of regimenting the meals, I like to have items that I can mix and match easily to create several different meals.

I'll give you some examples of what I regularly stock in my kitchen to give me a variety of anxiety-reducing options.

In the Pantry
+ Gluten-free all-purpose flour mix. This can be used for baking, sauces, coatings, etc. I *think* that's the point of the label "all purpose."
+ Gluten-free chicken stock (liquid or powder form). I make soup or use it as a base for many sauces. I also use this instead of water when making quinoa and rice to liven up some flavor. I use stock as a base for stir-fry too!
+ Coconut oil, olive oil, and/or other vegetable oils for cooking and baking. I suggest buying a mister so you can use olive oil for safe cooking. Avoid any baking sprays like PAM, as they might have flour in them.

✦ Canned coconut milk (I'm telling you now to go for the full-fat version. The low-fat milk is kinda like eating a low-fat donut). I use coconut milk to make easy Thai stir-fry dishes. You can also make breakfast quinoa with coconut milk in the rice cooker.

✦ Gluten-free baking mixes like brownies, pancakes, cakes and cupcakes. Brands like King Arthur Flour, Pamela's Products, Wholesome Chow, and XO Baking Co. make it easy to recreate gluten-free versions of your favorite gluten treats.

✦ Spices. Spices in their natural forms are gluten free and can liven up any boring dish. Buy expensive and organic spices; they will last a long time, and they are worth the extra expense! I like to keep these dried spices on hand at all times: kosher salt, black pepper, lemon pepper, rosemary, basil, dried minced garlic, garlic salt, dried onions, red pepper flakes, curry spice mixes, cinnamon, and pumpkin pie mix (or just straight-up cardamom if you're a baller because that shit is expensive).

✦ Sriracha. Duh.

✦ Gluten-free oats. Note that oats are often cross-contaminated with gluten, so purchase certified gluten free *only!* Also, even gluten-free oats can cause issues, so use in small amounts only until you've tried to see how sensitive you are to them.

✦ Unsalted or unflavored nuts for quick protein.

✦ Red and white quinoa to substitute for rice in dishes for more protein and to mix things up.

✦ Spaghetti sauce and pizza sauce. Make sure these sauces are gluten free and not made on the same equipment as wheat. The Classico brand is easy to find, and I think it's a great-quality brand.

✦ Gluten-free pretzels. We're addicted to Glutino, Snyder's gluten-free, and Gratify brands and are often found at mass retailers.

✦ Soup. You never know when you're going to get sick and not want to leave the couch. I always stock some gluten-free chicken noodle soup (usually found at natural markets). While major soup brands do have some gluten-free options, always check the label.

In the Freezer

+ Unflavored or unaltered fresh meat products such as ground turkey (Jennie-O products are happily labeled gluten free), ground beef, salmon and chicken.
+ Sausages are easy to cut up and add with anything in a stir-fry. We like Applegate Farms and Trader Joe's brands. Be careful— some sausages contain gluten!
+ Frozen vegetables without sauce. Go for the plain veggies, as some of the veggies in sauces contain gluten (on top of a ton of unnecessary ingredients too).
+ Ice cream or nondairy ice cream—like Rice Dreams, or Almond Dreams that are labeled gluten free.
+ Gluten-free pre-prepared cookie dough is great for quick desserts and the ability to make just a few cookies at a time. We dig the vegan gluten-free Eat Pastry chocolate chip dough, but there are plenty of other safe options including the mainstream brand Pillsbury!

In the Refrigerator

+ Fresh vegetables and fresh fruit should always be kept in stock for easy accessibility and a healthy gluten-free diet. Visit your local farmer's market for the freshest and in-season varieties.
+ Milk (or nondairy milk if you're like me. I like rice milk, almond milk, soy milk—although it makes me gassy—and hemp milk).
+ Spread, sauces, and butter. I prefer Earth balance nondairy butter spreads (because I can't have dairy frequently—mmmm-mmmm butter).
+ Tamari sauce or gluten-free soy sauce.

✦ Gluten-free curry paste. Don't be afraid—if I can make curry at home, so can you.

✦ Gluten-free salad dressings (or just olive oil and balsamic vinegar, which typically don't need to be refrigerated).

But what happens when you don't have a good gluten-free resource near you where you can buy these products?

1. **Subscription boxes.** If you don't have a Whole Foods or gluten-free specialty store near you, get items shipped to you! But, how do you order something you've never tasted before? Several companies have launched subscription-box services that feature various gluten-free products delivered monthly to your door. Gfreely, Taste Guru, Healthy Surprise, Tasterie, G-Free Foodie Box Club are some of the boxes that I've had experience with.

2. **Order online!** Amazon.com, Vitacost.com and The Gluten-Free Mall on Celiac.com are all great sources for gluten-free online shopping. You can also visit the website of any major gluten-free manufacturer and order directly from them. These brands will often send discount coupons to you if you sign up on their mailing list.

My last piece of advice to you is to branch out—try new brands, try new food, just try something out of the ordinary. If you've never tried making Thai food—branch out. Google a gluten-free recipe and get some new grocery items! Remember, you can always rely on gluten-free bloggers to give you the heads-up on great new gluten-free finds that you can scour your grocery store for too!

Gluten-Free Traveling—How to Survive the Unknown Outside Your Comfort Zone

I was never good at flying—in fact, I went to an anxiety specialist for my fear of it. Now, after years of flying for business, I'm used to it and very rarely have panic attacks while flying. However, traveling gluten free really threw a wrench in it. How was I going to stay safe in the airport, on the plane, or at the destination?

The answer is really only about preparedness. You always have to be prepared with gluten-free food—either bringing your own, and/or thoroughly researching your destination.

My number-one rule of gluten-free travel is to always err on the side of caution. This typically means I bring way too much food, and leave the destination with most of it still packed in my suitcase. But, you never know when you are going to have to resort to the food you brought instead of risking your health on unsafe food.

If you're traveling to your destination by car, it's easier because you can pack your car full of anything you may need. You can carry a cooler full of perishables until you reach your destination. You can use your own transportation to stock up at grocery stores and pit stops along the way and during your travels. Just make sure your final destination has a refrigerator to stock your perishables upon arrival!

Traveling by plane is a *bit* more difficult. I always pack at least two bags. One bag will hold all of my fabulous vintage outfits, and an extra bag or suitcase will be full of gluten-free food. If you can afford extra baggage fees, check the extra suitcase just for food. Just make sure that the suitcase is sturdy enough to get through rough baggage handling without its contents being crushed.

You just never know when you're going to have turn to your luggage-turned-pantry because you can't find anything safe. Or, if you're like me, you *need* a gluten-free cookie after dinner, and God knows where you're going to find those on your adventures in an unknown city.

Things to pack in your checked baggage:

+ Loaf of gluten-free shelf-stable bread and toaster bags[38]
+ Full jar of peanut butter or other nut butter packed full of protein
+ Squeezable baby food/fruit packets (I like HappyFamily brand)
+ Gluten-free protein mix (like Vega One or Nutrasumma) and a shaker for easy-to-make meal-replacement shakes
+ Gluten-free jerky for on-the-go protein—just be careful as many meat snacks have soy sauce in them (look for gluten-free brands like KRAVE or Shelton's)
+ Packets of gluten-free instant oatmeal (Bakery on Main or Glutenfreeda) that you can make using any hotel room's coffee pot
+ Gluten-free treats like cookies and brownies—even if you find a safe meal on the road or at an event, rarely do they also stock gluten-free desserts, so bring your own

---

[38] Toaster bags are small packages that you can put gluten-free bread into and use another toaster safely without cross-contamination. They also make awesome grilled cheese sandwiches out of your toaster! These are available to purchase online at Amazon.com.

During your travels, bring food that you wouldn't mind eating in lieu of a meal. Remember: *one cannot survive on gluten-free cookies alone.*

Due to the three-ounce TSA regulations, not much that's tasty can get through. Pack everything in your checked luggage that you may think could be considered a liquid. Even chunky peanut butter is considered a liquid—and tossing out an artisan jar of new nut butter is enough to make you shed a tear in security. And unless you have a spare baby on you, you'll need to pack those squeeze bags of applesauce and fruit too.

But what about before you even get to your destination? You never know when there will be airport delays for an ungodly amount of time. Pack more food than you think you will need in your carry-on luggage—both ways! I've had delayed flights happen too many times before. It seems to always happen when I'm not prepared—a four-hour delay at night when the restaurants are closed and/or the only thing to eat is McDonald's (a.k.a. there's still nothing safe to eat). Try to carry protein and hearty food that can tide you over through a long flight or a long wait (hopefully not both).

Things to pack in your carry-on luggage:

+ Empty water bottle so you can avoid high-priced bottled water after the security checkpoints, and stay hydrated during your trip
+ Protein-packed bars (Larabars, Pure Fruit & Nut bars, and KIND bars are my favorites)
+ Small squeeze packs of nut butter in your liquids bag (or not, if you can sweet-talk the TSA agent to letting it pass)
+ Premade sandwich like a nut butter that won't go bad if not refrigerated (unlike a turkey sandwich, unless you plan on eating as soon as you get to the airport)
+ Fresh washed and chopped fruit in plastic bags—making it easy to eat on the plane without having seeds, pits or peels left over with nowhere to toss your trash

Also, a must for your carry-on luggage is medications and digestive enzymes. The last thing you want to do on a plane is to feel like dog poop.

+ Since I'm sensitive to dairy and a few other items, I bring digestive enzymes with me wherever I go. Although these will not help anyone with celiac disease to eat gluten (because cheating is always a no-no), they can potentially help if you get accidentally cross-contaminated during your trip.

+ I use Tummy Drops and Gin-Gin brands of ginger candies to keep my wits about me if I get nauseated or uncomfortable on the plane.

When you get to your destination, you can refer back to the dining-out chapter and go from there. Utilize social media like Yelp and gluten-free dining apps to find the safest place for you to dine. Don't be afraid of taking a taxi or local transportation in order to reach a great (and safe) location; it will be worth the extra expense!

Gluten-free traveling for the first time can be scary and anxiety producing—especially if you already have an anxiety disorder like I do! But, like most things about the gluten-free lifestyle, it gets easier over time. You can't allow your fear of gluten to take over all aspects of your life. Tell gluten who is boss—and travel without fear knowing that you're prepared. You'll eventually learn how to properly pack for each occasion and navigate the sometimes-scary world outside of your front door!

The Power of Support:
Support Groups

I have to admit that I didn't go to my first celiac support group until I was a few years into my diagnosis. I kept putting it off, thinking that my stressful research job was too important to make friends and share in the gluten-free community. If I didn't even have time for the gym, how on earth would I find time to go to a support group? I wasn't an alcoholic; it's not like I needed a group of people to keep me 100% gluten free—I was already doing that on my own. I didn't have to make amends to anyone I had hurt during my gluten relapses (although sometimes I think I should apologize for being a monster when I snuck in gluten before I *knew* about cross-contamination). Why did I need someone else?

It was hard for me to take a few hours out to go to meetings. But looking back, that was all *so silly*. Where else could I go to meet a group of like-minded weird specialty dieters? Where else could I get a room full of celiacs together? What other opportunities would I have to learn from people just like me, living in the same geographical space as I was? Seriously, I was missing out.

Support groups are often run by local chapter volunteers of a national organization like Celiac Disease Foundation, Gluten Intolerance Group, or Celiac Sprue Association. These various national entities have local support groups spread throughout the US.

These support-group meetings are typically free to attend, but you should really think about donating or becoming a member. For my support group it is $40 to become a member of both the Celiac Disease Foundation national organization and the local chapter. On the local level, there are several benefits ranging from a packet of catalogs from companies that specialize in GF foods, information on living the GF lifestyle, lending privileges in the library of resources on GF living, voting privileges and the ability to serve as an officer. Being a member supports your local group's goals of celiac awareness and support in your area. On a national level, I receive perks from the national organization like newsletters and research updates. I really wanted to join because I believe in the organization, much like I believe in the other national foundations and organizations aimed at advancing research and raising awareness for celiac disease.

My first meeting was inclusionary, comforting and pretty enlightening. We've met so many amazing people at both support groups that we've attended. Just listening to their stories about diagnosis and life before the gluten-free fad-diet time was fascinating. We had a chance to meet members who spanned the entire spectrum of gluten sensitivity. Members also ranged in age of diagnosis—from those diagnosed with celiac when they were very young to those not diagnosed until middle age or later. It was so interesting to see people who had been living gluten free before they had access to so many packaged goods and had to make every gluten-free item from scratch. I'm *pretty* sure that I would have just wasted away if I didn't have dry mixes available to me with the ingredients portioned out just right. It made me feel incredibly lucky that I was diagnosed during the time period I was.

Non-GFBF and I spent a lot of time afterwards talking to members and meeting new fresh faces. I met a "younger person"[39] who just

---

[39] That was my nice way of saying that I met someone my age instead of someone in their 60s or 70s. Yeah, my group is full of old people—I'm okay with admitting that. But keep in mind that ages vary group to group and state to state.

moved to Arizona and was newly-diagnosed. It was so cathartic to see someone who was where I was when I was first diagnosed and to be able to provide some advice to help her along the way.

You can find your local chapter by visiting Celiac.org (Celiac Disease Foundation's website), Gluten.net (Gluten Intolerance Group's website), or CSAceliacs.info (Celiac Sprue Association's website). What do you do if you don't have a chapter near you? Work with one of these great organizations to found one for your community (but more on that later in the book).

Do you have family members who just don't understand your new lifestyle? Does someone you know not take you seriously when you talk about how important your diet is? Invite them to come to a meeting with you. Introduce them to other gluten-free people, and show them that this lifestyle is very important to you and your health.

Volunteer with these support group chapters, and you'll have an additional chance to meet others and work with the community. For example, our chapter puts on a gluten-free expo every year. I volunteered doing marketing for one of their events, and I loved working with them! It's a lot of work, but it's worth giving back to the gluten-free community that you are a part of—kudos!

Be sure to organize play dates outside of the meetings. Go out for dinner and try new safe restaurants. This can be a time to leave the significant other behind so you can talk realistically (and privately) about living life gluten free.

One of the organizations we work with gathers gluten-free food every meeting and donates to a local food bank. Many food banks do not offer gluten-free menu items, as they simply do not have enough of it). If you belong to a chapter and don't have this program going, I'm asking you, yes you, to start this at your chapter. Find someone to be the designated food-bank liaison, and they can collect and then donate the gluten-free shelf-stable food that is collected. Don't have a group but still interested in this? Call your local food bank and ask if you can start a program in your community to donate gluten-free food and work with local gluten-free-friendly grocers to run a food drive!

Support groups also help to highlight local vendors. Groups will typically feature local safe businesses or national vendors that produce gluten-free items. Not only will you meet friends, but you can discover new food while you're at it! Also, many groups will have special events where support-group members can bring their own homemade treats and have recipe exchanges. I've found plenty of new recipes from fellow support group members.

In my opinion, libraries are also an important part of support groups. These books are typically donated by the author or purchased using fundraising dollars. At our groups, you can "rent" the book and return it at the next meeting. This is a great opportunity to get a look inside new cookbooks before buying them.

If you're not able to make meetings or don't want to venture outside your comfort zone, there are plenty of online support groups. I am a member of two online Facebook support groups for celiac disease (as well as some for other concurrent conditions). These groups are founded and moderated by well-known gluten-free bloggers, and are no-holds-barred and full of the raw emotions of living a gluten-free life. If you're not happy with the content you've found online, head over to these groups and connect with others that surely feel *just like you*. There are also online communities run by major gluten-free brands, but the content is often moderated strictly by the brand and not as intimate as other groups.

Regardless of how you find support, please seek it out. You'll meet people like you and find comfort in finally being just. like. everyone. else. For once. You don't have to face the gluten-free world alone!

Gluten-Free Expos:
How to Shove Grocery Bags
Full of Free Food in Suitcases

Going to an expo, conference, or convention that is focused on safe gluten-free *only* foods is a real treat—like a Christmas where you unwrap every gift and get everything you want. You step into a hall filled with foods—and can eat anything there without having to read countless ingredients (assuming you're not allergic to additional items besides gluten, although there are many dairy-free, soy-free and other things-free options there too).

My first expo was overwhelming, much like my first "anything" experience after going gluten free. There were so many new products out there; I grabbed every coupon I saw and stuffed my face with every product available. It was like I had walked into Willy Wonka's chocolate factory and I just wanted to bathe myself in everything gluten free. If you've ever taken children to Disneyland, it's a lot like that. By the end of the day, I felt just as bloated, nauseated and worn out as a five-year old who was slammed with an eight-hour immersion into everything Mickey Mouse and fair food. It was exhausting, but it's so worth it.

Who attends these magical events? Bloggers are there as press to report back on the newest products, but also to meet their readers and gain new followers. Manufacturers of gluten-free brands will be there to introduce their product to new users. Hopefully if their product is yummy they will actually have it for sale so I can buy it! Big brands also give out awesome swag like chip clips, magnets, or t-shirts. Gluten-free and celiac organizations will be there to help you along your journey (and sign you up for a membership, which I recommend). And the average, everyday consumer? We are there to eat to our hearts' content! We want to taste every new product out there and get excited about all the new stuff we have to eat!

There are plenty of other gluten-free expos out there—many that I've had the pleasure to attend over the years. Some are small parties, while some are huge expos of more than 5,000 people. Jen Cafferty, of the popular Gluten & Allergen Free Expo, puts on phenomenal expos. I like them because they are huge, they tackle major cities, and they are friendly to many allergies on top of gluten. I've been an official blogger for them in the past, and now I'm an official vendor. I encourage everyone I meet to visit an expo of hers. Wherever you go, make sure that you inquire about the expo and how vendors are approved. You want to make sure that the vendors involved with the event are quality vendors that are truly gluten-free so you can have the best (and safest) experience possible.

After tackling a handful of different expos over the past few years, I've accumulated several tips for those who haven't yet been to a gluten-free event.

Be outgoing, even if you have to fake it. Sometimes it's hard for me to be at an event talking to strangers all day. Even though I appear very outgoing, sometimes events like this are too much for me. I really have to psych myself up to be in a huge crowd where I'll have to introduce myself a thousand times and attempt to remember that many names. If you're anything like me, these events can be overwhelming due to sheer size. Do some deep-breathing exercises, and put your game face on! Now is the time to reach out and connect, so don't risk that just to be a wallflower!

Connect with others. These events are not just about food. Take time to meet the fellow expo attendees who live in your area. Now is the time to connect with future gluten-free friends! Haven't you wanted to find someone to go with to all the new restaurants that you've been dying to try? Reach out and make a connection to someone you've never met and make a new GFF (gluten-free friend).

Why connect? Just like in the support-group chapter, you need to know that there are people like you out there. It's positive to see people thrive with the same condition you have. It's cathartic to share experiences and meet someone with the same situations you face every day.

Wear comfortable shoes. You're going to be walking a *lot* around the expo hall. I have known only one person who can wear high heels all day, and I attribute that trait to being a super hero, not an average person (you know who you are, Kyra). Wear tennis shoes or comfortable loafers (like Toms)—something to make the day comfortable.

Pack an extra suitcase. If you're coming in from out of town, make sure you pack an extra TSA-approved carry-on bag along with your checked suitcase. You'll need the extra room to stash all of your goodies and swag from the expo! If you live locally this is less of an issue, because you can take home all of the goodies in your car. If you live locally and the expo is a two-day event, go both days and stock up on the freebies, as well as spend more time talking in-depth to each vendor. It's really awesome to get a chance to talk to a representative from your favorite company (or maybe your least favorite too) and give feedback or props to them in person!

Eat a full meal. I've seen too many bloggers tell people to come to expos hungry. While I believe that it is important to have room in your stomach to snack, you should really eat a full meal before attending. If you just rely on cookies, crackers, or other items typically found at expos, your blood sugar might get wonky—and no one wants that. Eat a protein so you can stay nourished while you indulge in treats and small snacks at the expo.

Don't feel pressure. There will be *plenty* of samples available. Some might even say that you wouldn't be able to eat them all even if you wanted to. Don't feel pressure to eat everything you see there! If there is a snack that doesn't look inviting, or you're too full, it's okay to politely decline it. If you're interested in the product but too full, take some of their literature or coupons so you can let the brand know that you are still interested and want to sample the product at a later time. If they offer pre-packaged samples, ask to take another one so you can try the product again at another time. Also, if there's a product you will never try, don't feel pressure to take their literature or coupons if you aren't going to use them.

Drink plenty. And no, I don't just mean gluten-free beer. You're going to be walking around for a while, so stay hydrated with water. Bring a thermos or water bottle so you can easily refill it throughout the event. And if you *are* planning on drinking alcohol at the event, be responsible. Where's the fun in sampling food if you can't remember what all you ate afterwards?

Bring digestive enzymes. Although all the manufacturers should be safe—as most are vetted before they become a vendor—you never know when something could make you feel like crap. For me, I always overdo it on the dairy, so I make sure to bring lots of natural digestive enzymes like papaya tablets with me. Also, I've heard that activated charcoal works as well for accidental exposure based on purely anecdotal evidence from fellow sensitive people (but always research potential adverse side effects).

Bring a pen. You'll want to make notes on vendor literature or business cards. Bring a pen or a sharpie (pencils might not work on card stock material). Did a chocolate chip cookie just blow your mind? Do you want to remember to *never* buy that product again? Make a note on the card so you can remember after your post-expo food coma. If there are seminars and education events during the event, make sure you bring a pen and paper so you can take notes. Even if the presenters will be putting their slides up online afterwards, oftentimes they'll give additional tidbits of important information that isn't included in the presentation. If you are a blogger or have a blog or website, bring enough business cards to give to all of the vendors.

Take pictures. I get so overwhelmed with all the sights, sounds, and smells of the expo that I'll forget about some products the next day. I take pictures of my favorite foods or companies. Also, you'll probably have a chance to meet and greet some key bloggers, gluten-free celebs and authors. You'll definitely want to have a camera for those photographic moments for future Facebook envy! Don't forget to share pics of the latest new products with fellow celiacs!

Bring cash. On top of free samples, many vendors will sell their products at expos. Expos give you an opportunity to purchase products that you might not be able to find at your local grocery store. Even in Phoenix—a bustling metropolitan city with lots of gluten-free options and grocery stores—I still find new products at expos and spend my cash on lots of new yummies. Gluten-free food is constantly reinventing itself. Products are getting better all the time. You will want to take this chance to stock up on items or buy new products. Some vendors take credit cards, so bring your Visa, but also bring cash in case some vendors take only cold hard cash.

I love the food, the people and the safe environment of these gluten-free events and expos. At events like this, you're not the *only* one who is sick, you're not the *only* one who has to read labels, you're not the *only* one excited about the latest bread on the market, and you're not the *only* one who hangs on every update regarding new gluten-free research. You can really be *you*—and that's a powerful thing to be!

What's Next: How to Be a Gluten-Free Advocate

———

Okay, so you've now read most of the book (either that or you cheated and totally skipped ahead to this chapter). Hopefully you have a better grasp of how I live gluten free, and perhaps you've learned a thing or two about how *you* can lead a better gluten-free life. So what's next? Oh, you know, *just living the rest of your entire life here on earth gluten free*. It's just that simple (insert laughter here).

Sometimes things are really hard for me still—even years after going gluten free. I still struggle on a weekly basis. Some weeks are better than others, and some days are better than others. But I couldn't keep feeling sorry for myself and I couldn't keep crying over spilled milk (and crumbs of gluten). Sooner or later I had to embrace this lifelong lifestyle change (and you do too if you haven't already).

This is who I am now, and I'm deciding to take the high road about it. I'm deciding to be proud. So when days get tough, I'm going to try to stay positive. I'm not going to sugarcoat my life—but when days get hard, I'm going to go down swinging. I'm not going to give up on celiac disease; I'm going to spend every day fighting—fighting for awareness, fighting to find positivity in this lifestyle, and fighting to change how a gluten-free lifestyle is perceived.

I came up with my new mantra to keep in mind when the going gets tough and wheat-y.

I never want my illness to define me, but since it's with me forever, I've learned to live with it and embrace it. It's always a positive point of conversation—about the power of being healthy and the power of food. I'm allowing celiac to make me a more interesting person—not a burden, and no longer the "sick" girl. I am an advocate, not a victim. Some days get me down, but days like today I feel proud that I'm taking control of my body.

It may take you years to feel the way that I do about celiac disease, or you may never feel the same. You may just want to live a quiet, gluten-free life removed from the community. Food may be a personal issue to you, and you may not want to put yourself out there and become an advocate. That's perfectly fine with me (as long as you're not cheating when doing so). But, this is the only way I could move from a diagnosis on to something positive.

I realized that I had a voice, but at the time I just didn't know what to do with it. Here's a post from my Facebook page in December 2011.

> *Just wrote an incredibly long and incredibly disjointed email to a mom whose little girl (who also has Down syndrome) just got diagnosed with celiac disease. I had no idea how much advice I had until I wrote it all down. I hope I can mentor them and help her out. Should I run one of those annoying food-allergy blogs? I feel annoying with or without wheat.*

How little did I know then just *how* annoying I could be! The world was my oyster!

I started *Celiac and the Beast* because I wanted my voice out there. I relied on bloggers when I was first diagnosed, and I wanted to give back to the community. I also saw that there was a white space in the blogosphere—room for a sarcastic "real" blogger who can be open about struggles (and open about success too). Sometimes it's nice to hear the real struggles of living life gluten free; it just makes it seem so humanizing, *so real*. I don't understand how some bloggers are just puppies and sunshine all the time! How do you have time to make all of your own meals to avoid being glutened? How do you prepare pasta from scratch so you don't have to deal with manufacturers and whether or not their facility-cleaning procedures are proper? How do you feed your kids when all they want is gluten-filled cupcakes? How are there no struggles in your life? I don't even have kids, but man, I struggle daily. *That's reality, but so is my choice to try to find the inspiration in crappy situations and opportunities to learn and teach from them as well.*

If you've reached the point in your gluten-free path where you'd like to become a part of the community, here are my suggestions for getting involved.

Get involved in the community: First, visit support groups and feel out which group best matches your wants and needs. Support groups (like I mentioned in a previous chapter) can be very different from each other. Before committing to a group, go to a few meetings at different groups and feel them out. Once you have found a group or groups that you like, volunteer and get involved! Help out with events and expos. Help organize special meetings. For example, our group puts on a special meeting once a year that features local restaurants and local chefs that do GF properly for a Q&A about dining out gluten free. Join the board, and recruit new members to join the support group. You'll feel like a part of the community and also help others grow along their own gluten-free path.

Go to events: Visit MeetUp.com and find a gluten-free event in your area. Bookmark GlutenFreeCalendar.com on your web browser for an ever-growing list of gluten-free events across the country. Check local support groups' websites and Facebook pages for meetings, events, and group outings. If there isn't already a strong presence in your community, encourage local gluten-free restaurants or bakeries to host GF meet-ups and events at their location.

Start a movement: So far, do all of these things sound super awesome, but they're not in your area? Well, then start something yourself! If you feel alone in your community, there's a chance that others do as well. If you have more than 200 people living in your town, there's a chance you're not the only celiac there—and at least a handful of gluten-intolerant folks too! Your movement could be anything! You could start your own chapter of the CDF, GIG or CSA in your area if you don't already have one. To organize that, you'll have to connect with the corresponding national organizations. You could also start a MeetUp.com group. Publicize your group on Facebook and at local gluten-free bakeries and restaurants. Ask local gluten-free businesses to sponsor your group with basic needs and sponsored treats during meetings in exchange for advertising. However you can put it together, just find a group of people like you, and celebrate friendships and safe eating.

Start your *own* blog: I've had many people ask how to start their own blogs. I think the biggest recommendation is just to go for it. However, when I mean "go for it," I really mean, "work your ass off." Although I do believe you can have a full-time job *and* a family and be a blogger—it will be difficult. You'll have to work on your blog when you're not busy working and not busy being a wife or mother. You'll have to find time on your own where you can actually sit down and spill out your thoughts onto the keyboard. I often get asked, "How do you do it all?" The only answer I can give them is about sacrificing. Right now, Non-GFBF is sitting on the couch watching a movie, and I'm on the couch typing away. Yes, I'm paying attention to the movie, but I've found a way to multi-task—and that's the only way I'm able to have a somewhat social life and be able to keep up with *Celiac and the Beast*. There are approximately one million unread CATB e-mails in my inbox about new products that companies want me to try, or companies following up with reviews or requests for something. I am terrible at reading and returning e-mails on time, which is not a good trait for any blogger. But, I'm putting niceties on hold while I try to finish this book. Hopefully all of these brands will give me a little break by the time I get back into the game.

Here are some things I *beg* of you when you start your own blog:

1. **Don't spread false information.** Oh dear God, how much I *hate* this. When you repost information, make sure it's from credible sources like the University of Chicago Celiac Disease Center, Celiac Disease Foundation, or National Foundation for Celiac Awareness. There are too many businesses and groups out there that like to propagate false information and scare tactics.

2. **Don't be sensational.** This is something I can't stand in the news media, and something I despise from bloggers too. Every post starts with "Is there really gluten in XYZ?" or "Could you be poisoning yourself and not even know it?" or something equally as terrifying. Basically, they post scare tactics to get you to read their articles, which may or may not actually contain facts or something worth reading. Aren't we all scared enough of everything? We don't need more nightmares when we already dream nightly about donuts. Yes, coffee, corn, and wine are all safe. Please continue living your life now.

3. **Don't pit readers against each other in a game of "who is sicker."** It's such a shame to see this in the autoimmune community. Since the symptoms of our type of condition vary, instead of people trying to console others with a "Don't worry you're not alone" attitude, it can sometimes turn into an "Oh yeah? *My* symptoms are worse" type of conversation.

I often feel like I am not good enough to be a gluten-free blogger because I don't suffer as bad as others when I am glutened. However, recent research states that the amount or severity of symptoms don't necessarily equate to the degree of damage. That's insane! It's crazy talk that I don't feel "good enough" because I'm not sick enough when I compare myself to others. We shouldn't have to compare horror stories to see who has it worse. No one wins in that scenario.

Although you may not start posts with the intention of leading people into a competition, if you see it happening—head it off at the start. We all suffer—and regardless of how *much* we suffer, we still need a supportive community.

Stay Humble: When I started my website, I thought maybe I'd have a few followers: definitely my mom, probably a few people from the support group, and maybe a few people who found me from Google. I was very excited when my numbers increased—and kept increasing. But, I have to realize that although I provide a service (free support and nonmedical advice on living gluten free), I'm just a girl with celiac disease—and that's all I can be. And that's who we all are—just people, facing a life free of gluten.

I used to think that these bloggers with hundreds of thousands of followers were these untouchable deities in the interwebs. But, after meeting some of them, I realized that they are just amazing people with amazing writing skills. They aren't very different from you and me—just people faced with a diagnosis, a mission, and a MacBook.

Everyone who I've met that I've considered "a celebrity" has been incredibly humble, which makes me only love and respect them more. Even though they have thousands upon thousands of followers, they don't have big heads or big egos. Although I'm not really sure if there is such a thing as a celebrity blogger, it's probably better if you never think of yourself as one, even if you get called one. Stay humble and try not to get a big head if (or should I say when) you gain a following.

Don't expect to become rich off of a blog (or shirts, or books):
You can't expect to quit your job and live off your blog income. At least,
I sure couldn't at the time of this book's publication. If for some reason,
you're reading this book and I'm a millionaire, I probably just got lucky
at the casino. While I started my blog because I'd been laid off, I still
had an average income from freelancing. Although I'm so thankful for
some sort of income, I find it crazy that I've been out of a full-time job
for a year now, and I still haven't found a job. But, I guess that's another
book about how to survive unemployment without turning into the crazy
cat lady from *The Simpsons* (hey book publishers—*call me*).

While I make enough to keep the lights on and afford organic
vegan pizza at Whole Foods, I thought *maybe* I could earn a living
from advertising on my site. I mean, I was working my tail off, so why
wouldn't a company want to pay money to be on my website? Well, as
of the day I wrote this sentence, I was not getting paid money for *any*
of the ads on my site. I've signed up to be an affiliate (where I put up a
brand's ad, and if someone clicks through from the ad on my site *and*
makes a purchase, I get a percentage of the product sales) for several
sites, but I've never received any money. From a marketer's perspective, I
often feel like a failure because these brands that love to send me samples
don't buy my ad space. But, I haven't been focused on sales; I've been
focused on writing about my life and what I put in my mouth.

There are plenty of other gluten-free bloggers who get a ton of traffic
to their sites. I see their ad space, and I'm sure that they're getting businesses to pay for their 300x250 ad units. And I'm sure that those people
have amazing recipes and some may even have help running their site
or contributing to their blog. That's awesome, but that's not really me
right now, and I'm not sure if it ever will be. If a brand is going to buy
ad space on my site, they're going to buy it because they love me—and
my lack of kitchen skills and my sarcasm.

I started my clothing line out of sheer luck. Although we had
experimented with a few shirts we got for super cheap, we didn't do a

full launch until Christmas. Non-GFBF had been telling me for weeks that I was going to love my Christmas present more than any other Christmas present ever. I didn't believe him, because I love Christmas, and I'm used to getting some pretty amazing gifts from him. I opened up a small box and started to cry. Inside was a set of multi-colored stickers of different gluten-free-themed designs he created for me and CATB. Not only did he create stickers, but he designed a custom-made hooded sweatshirt that featured our now infamous Gluten Free For Life skull design. As soon as I posted a picture of myself wearing the hoodie on Instagram, it was a hit. We experimented with some shirt and hoodie designs based on my very popular Christmas gift, and the rest is history (and available for sale on my website!).

Although I make a profit off of every shirt and hooded sweatshirt we sell, there are expos and events where I barely break even. Our profits go back into stocking more product and travel costs to attend multiple expos across the country. I would love to be able to travel the world with this book, some shirts, and my smile without relying on a day job, but as of right now I don't see that happening. But who knows, maybe I'll marry rich one day?

So, if you read this book to try to figure out how to get rich from blogging, I'm sorry but you've come to the wrong place.

I'm just a girl. Writing about being gluten free in a world full of wheat.

I'm just trying to make the process easier for everyone. I'm just trying to help you learn to love the beast—or at least learn to live with it. Over the past few years, I can only hope to have made a difference in someone's life. I found my calling and my passion—being the voice for other gluten-free folks who don't have one. I hope you can do the same if you are passionate about this community.

The End: Burned Bits and Acknowledgements

I think the tastiest parts of gluten-free baked goods often come from the burned bits that fall just outside the muffins onto the baking pans. These bits are the first thing that I eat when I pull the pan out of the oven because each one is unique and interesting, unlike its muffin brethren. These little bits had the nerve to do something a little outside the lines and probably outside their muffin comfort zone.

Writing this book, I tried to focus on the burned bits—the stories and advice a little outside the lines when it comes to writing a gluten-free lifestyle book. I tried to let my unique personality and sense of humor shine through, so you could relate to the struggles and celebrations of someone living a life much like yours. Because living life gluten free isn't all perfectly formed muffins, puppies and sunshine, as you've clearly read.

My life has changed dramatically since my diagnosis. Often I think that it has changed for the *better*—although some days I still want to punch celiac in the face. But, it has definitely changed me, and I hope that it can change you. I hope living a gluten-free life can create a healthier and happier version of you. I hope that you find love and support in this lifestyle and find a way to adapt with ease. I hope I can get you to learn to love the beast, or at least learn to live with it.

My friend Kim asked if she could write the foreword to my book. Since I didn't have a foreword, I'm putting her praise here.

> *"Here is everything you need to know. Erica is f-cking rad. Enjoy this labor of love, coffee, and non-gluten."*

I thought it summed up my thoughts pretty well. I've really put a lot of myself into this book, and I hope to God someone finds it as *rad* as Kim thinks *I* am.

Who would I like to thank for this labor of love?

My parents. Of course! They gave me life, so why wouldn't I acknowledge them here? My parents are both amazing humans. Mostly because they created me—celiac and all! Thank you for your support throughout all of this—sickness to diagnosis to starting my own gluten-free blog to writing this book. Thank you for always believing in me, regardless of what I choose to do. God knows I'm still trying to figure out who I want to be when I grow up!

Non-GFBF (aka Matt). He deserves to be acknowledged for being the most amazing life partner I've had (okay, I've only had one but he's really awesome). Matthew, I love you with all of my heart, except the part that is reserved for reality television and donuts and wine. I can't thank you enough for the past few years. It speaks volumes on the type of man that you are that you're willing to put up with my shenanigans on a regular basis. Also, I'm really glad that you're a talented graphic designer, because I hear it's pretty expensive to have someone design a website and an entire apparel line.

My doctors. I'd especially like to thank the docs at Mayo Clinic and Dr. Lucinda Harris for figuring out what the hell was wrong with me.

Everyone who contributed on Kickstarter. If you donated $1 or $500, I am beyond thankful to all of you for helping make this dream a reality! I appreciate all of your support throughout this process.

My friends. I am so thankful for my friendships—especially those that have pushed me harder than I've pushed myself on getting this book done. Often during this process, they believed in me more than I've believed in myself. I was overwhelmed with the outpouring of love and encouragement from my Facebook friends. Sometimes I forget that I'm actually posting stuff that people can see—so thank you for all the likes, positive comments, and sharing my Kickstarter campaign with your friends and family. I really appreciate your support and not unfriending me when I post so many cat photos.

To Shauna—for keeping me writing, even when I didn't want to, and for your passion for gluten-free living (and you get major street cred for being GF before it was cool and before even I got diagnosed). To Kim—even though my first book idea was approximately a millennium ago and was about a completely different subject, you've always encouraged me to write. To Lisa J, Annette and Kristen—you have always taught me to put on my big-girl panties and go for what I want in life (without whining too much). Thank you ladies—you mean more to me than you know.

Gluten-Free Family. I have also met the most amazing group of bloggers and gluten-free advocates throughout my few years being online. I'd like to send some major gluten-free love out to these great people: Mary Fran from FrannyCakes, Chrissy from Glam Without Gluten, K.C. from G-Free Foodie, Alison from A Girl Defloured, Brandy Wendler, Kyra from Kyra's Bake Shop, Chandice from Gluten Free Frenzy, Ken from Rock a Healthy Lifestyle, Alysa from InspiredRD, Sarah from CanIEatHere.com, Rebecca from Pretty Little Celiac, Melissa from Geekily GF, Alissa from Breaking Up With Captain Crunch, and Gluten Dude. There are so many other amazing bloggers who are out there working their tails off spreading the word about gluten-free living. While I'm trying to keep my word count up, listing all of them would take up way too much space. Follow my social media, and you'll see that I repost a lot of their content. I share their content because these bloggers are amazing. Taking time out of your life to serve others and help advocate for the community makes these people extraordinary.

Thank you for all of your support.